MW00461770

# Fire Your Narrator!

# Fire Your Narrator!

## A Storyteller's Guide to Getting Out of Your Head and Into Your Life

*by*
**Valerie Gordon**

Copyright © 2021 Valerie Gordon

All rights reserved. No part of this publication may be reproduced, distributed, or transmitted in any form or by any means, including photocopying, recording, or other electronic or mechanical methods, without the prior written permission of the publisher, except in the case of brief quotations embodied in critical reviews and certain other noncommercial uses permitted by copyright law. For permission requests, write to the publisher, addressed "Attention: Permissions Coordinator," at the address below.

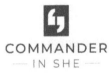

COMMANDER
— IN SHE —

https://commander-in-she.com

ISBN: 978-1-7374345-0-4 (print)
ISBN: 978-1-7374345-1-1 (ebook)

Ordering Information:
Special discounts are available on quantity purchases by corporations, associations, and others. For details, contact info@commander-in-she.com

*This book is for anyone in need of a
better story.*

*And for my mother, the best writer
I know.*

# TABLE OF CONTENTS

# TABLE OF CONTENTS

# FOREWORD

## BY MATTHEW DICKS

On July 12, 2011, I took to the stage in New York City and told the story of my life for the first time to an audience of strangers. It was a Moth StorySLAM – a storytelling competition – that I had entered on the urging of my friends who thought I had stories worth sharing. My plan was to tell one story, check "storytelling" off my bucket list, and never perform again.

Instead, I won that first StorySLAM and have gone on to win many more. More importantly, I found something that I loved and that has changed my life.

Since that first night in New York, I have traveled the world telling stories and teaching storytelling to every type of person and organization imaginable. Marketers and salespeople. Priests, minsters, and rabbis. Native Americans and Santa Clauses. Doctors and nurses. Grandparents and docents. Authors and poets. Teachers and professors. Advertising agencies. People looking to make friends and improve their dating prospects. Politicians hoping to win votes. Comedians trying to connect with their audiences.

The remarkable thing about storytelling is that no matter what you do, telling better stories will make you better at whatever you are. It will help you connect and communicate. It will draw people to you. It will help you convince others that your product, service, idea, or argument is good. It will cause people – sometimes total strangers – to share their deepest secrets with you.

So, I wrote a book on the subject: *Storyworthy: Engage, Teach, Persuade, and Change Your Life Through the Power of Storytelling.* My wife and I launched Speak Up, an organization dedicated to helping people find and tell their best stories. We began producing storytelling shows throughout New England in theaters, museums, art spaces, and more, growing our audience with each and every show. Thanks to Speak Up and my book, I began meeting remarkable storytellers from all over the world.

Best of all, I also learned from talented storytellers in my backyard and in our audience.

Valerie Gordon first came to Speak Up as an audience member and a lover of stories. She was still unknown to me when she pitched me a story about lying to Neil Diamond for our show themed "That's Weird." The story sounded interesting, so my wife and I invited Valerie to perform in an upcoming show. She was three sentences into her story when I knew that we had found a talented, skilled, experienced storyteller. Valerie immediately put me at ease with her confidence, her craft, her humor, and her pitch-perfect performance.

Our audience instantly fell in love with Valerie, and we've cast her in many shows since that first night. She never fails to impress.

Despite her talent, Valerie – like many performers – has a tendency to get into her head while performing or immediately after the performance is complete. You would never know it to listen to her tell a story, but she has that unfortunate impulse to think about what she did wrong as opposed to what went well.

It's surprisingly common for many storytellers. They tell these brilliant, inspiring, hilarious, heartfelt stories onstage while telling themselves decidedly less helpful stories that can stifle creativity and cast doubt in their minds.

It's surprising, at least to me, because I have somehow managed to avoid this mental pugilism. I am certainly capable of critiquing my performance, but I'm never hard on myself.

I suspect that an unbearable degree of confidence plays a role.

Unbearable confidence isn't always a great thing (just ask my wife), but I feel lucky. I can't imagine what it would be like to have a voice in my head constantly working against me. Performing onstage is hard enough already. Public speaking demands all of your energy and focus. For many, it takes an enormous amount of courage to stand alone onstage and speak. Taking the stage, saddled by a mind filled with criticism and self-doubt, only makes a hard thing exponentially harder. What purpose does that rotten little voice serve? More importantly, how do you silence it?

As a teacher of storytelling, Valerie's book is an invaluable resource to me. It's been difficult for me to help storytellers silence that inner critic when I've never been forced to silence my own. Not only does this book offer smart, actionable tips for those who need to fire their personal narrator, but it's fascinating to get a peek into a mind so different from my own and understand their thoughts better.

I plan on stealing all of Valerie's ideas and using them often.

You should, too.

# PROLOGUE

## THIS IS STUPID

### *Squash That Voice in Your Head*

This is stupid. I mean, like, really stupid.

Who's going to read a book I write? Who am I to think I can finish a book?

I tried twice before and bailed on both attempts. Why? Because of those little "nots" that keep me tied up in knots that seem impossible to unravel. Not focused enough. Not disciplined enough. Not talented enough. The furthest I got was to chapter 13 back in 2008 when I weighed 20 pounds less than I do now. That fact has nothing to do with anything, other than to cement the idea that my proposed shortcomings go far beyond my writing abilities. Not fit enough. Not pretty enough. Too old. Too late.

Who's going to read this anyway? I mean, really: Why are you here? Don't you have something better to do?

It's ironic that as I write a book about the powerful role of our inner narrator, that internal voice that guides our hopes and goals and dreams, I have an entirely unhelpful voice of my own getting in the way of my own hopes and goals and dreams. Who am I to tell you, the reader, how to manage that voice in your head when mine squashes my confidence with every sentence I write?

So that's what I call her. Squash. She's that voice in my head. Squash is a fitting name because her only purpose seems to be to squash me and keep me small. I picture her as some sort of evil Viking woman, always arguing, questioning, and scoring like a harsh Russian judge taking points off your perfect triple axel in the Olympics because you didn't smile upon landing. (Can you be both Viking and Russian? In my mind, she is.)

Squash is always with me, an invisible shadow in my brain, whispering in my ear. But instead of sweet nothings, Squash reminds me of my many shortcomings and offers such scathing sentiments as "This will never work," and "You totally screwed that up," and "Oh my god, did you just eat that ENTIRE BOX of Wheat Thins?"

It's Squash who assembles uninvited guests in my head at 3:30 in the morning when I wake with anxiety for a gathering I never intended to host (Chapter 19). It's Squash who reminds me of embarrassing memories I'd rather forget, like that breakfast meeting when I watched in horror as a tiny bit of spittle flew from my mouth and landed in the middle of the conference room table atop a platter of previously admired pastries that now included one lonely donut no one was going to touch (Chapter 7). That was years ago, and I still can't forget. Thanks, Squash.

And it's Squash who feeds me garbage when there's clearly healthier fare to chew on. I'm not talking about those Wheat Thins I can't resist once the box is open but the head trash that I recycle through my overthinking mind (Chapter 12). Squash always points out the worst in me while ignoring or negating the good. Who gave her such power? I did.

We all have an inner narrator. You have your own version of Squash living between your ears, narrating your day. It's a voice you've likely carried around since childhood that now offers future predictions like a bad movie trailer. You've likely never named the voice, as I've named Squash, because it's so much a part of you that you've just come to accept it as yourself. Although you know the voice is unhelpful, you don't know how to stop listening.

I don't recall when I first started speaking to myself in that squashing way. Maybe in fourth grade when I felt awkward and oversized, towering over my classmates and sporting both glasses and a mouthful of braces. Maybe in high school when a boy I liked regarded me with intensity one day, only to point out, "You have a giant zit on your nose." He was right. I did.

I do know that the voice became louder and more insistent over time. Squash is the one questioning, doubting, criticizing, and reviewing every failure or embarrassment. When things go well, as I've learned they often do, Squash reminds me I got lucky, or it was undeserved, or that good times never last so don't get too comfortable. She overemphasizes my insecurities much like a magnifying mirror exaggerates the size of my pores and the remnants of my ravaged teenage skin.

What – or who – is in *your* head? And ... why? Why would you create such a story?

I've made a living producing stories that educate, entertain, and inspire. I understand how three elements – character, plot, and narrative point of view – are essential to a story and how rising and falling actions create climax and resolution. Now I teach clients how to use the power of their own stories to advance their careers, improve their brand, get unstuck, and turn the page. But you can't tell a great external story if you're struggling with the internal one. It's why, even though you're the star of your own story, your inner narrator is by far the most influential character.

Character is who a story is about. In every best-selling paperback or romantic comedy, we root for the protagonist though she may be flawed or lacking. In fact, we prefer characters who are flawed. We see ourselves in them as complex beings in a challenging world. In your own story, it's OK if you're flawed or lacking. We root for you more that way, and frankly, we like you better. Those flaws make you authentic, relatable, and capable of growth and change. Show up as you are.

Plot is the action of the story. I don't care how boring you think your life is, something is happening. There are plot points created through choices and actions and twists and turns we didn't see coming that we respond to with more choices and actions. Conflict or challenge and how we respond to them are plot drivers. Because we are flawed and lacking, we don't always make the best choices, which leads to more conflict and additional challenges. That's what makes the story interesting! Think about it – you've never read, heard, or watched a story that didn't involve some type of conflict. We want to see the struggle before the success. And yet, in our own stories, who likes conflict? Who wants to struggle? No one! But that's what makes the story worthwhile and the success that much sweeter.

Both character (who we are, how we think of ourselves) and plot (what we do, how we proceed) are influenced by that third essential story element, our narrative point of view. In storytelling, the narrative point of view – or POV – is the voice or tone of the story. It's how the story is told and how it is received by the listeners. They, in turn, filter their story through their own point of view, which leads to all sorts of interpretation and, yes, more conflict.

It doesn't matter what actually happens in reality, because our narrator creates the narrative framework through which we view the world. Through that lens, we interpret experiences, prioritizing those that confirm our beliefs and ignoring those that don't. That framework affects our behaviors, actions, optimism, and relationship with ourselves and others. We use our memories of the past – our internal narrative – to guide us through present decisions. Our present decisions then create future impacts – the story of what comes *next*. That's why the narrator is the most important character in our own story. It colors our world and makes changing our perception and our future story difficult if not downright unlikely. You might second-guess yourself out of taking those chances or making positive choices. Will you raise your hand at the conference to ask that question (*or not, because it's probably stupid*), or cold-call for that potential opportunity (*or not, because really, what's the point?*), or eat the rest of that just-opened box of Wheat Thins? (*Might as well. That would be just like you, Fat Girl!*)?

Geez, Squash, stuff it!

Through my years of work, I've become fascinated by our own internal stories and how they impact our external results. In order to speak confidently of ourselves and create new opportunities, we have to recognize and rewrite internal stories that are old, outdated, or no longer serve us. When audiences and clients discover their own Squash, it's like switching on a light bulb after years of darkness and illuminating what they haven't previously been able to see. They understand the influence their inner narrator has held and how it's held them back.

Most people consider this voice an "inner critic," but as you'll see in this book (that Squash insists I'll never finish – check that, Squash; I'm jamming through this prologue!), the narrator plays many roles. A critical inner voice is the most familiar, but your personal narrator is a unique combination of experiences and stories you've reaffirmed for yourself over time. It's a voice from the past, along for the ride in the present and keeping a chokehold on your future.

If you've got a narrator like Squash, know that you *can* recast the voice with a better and more productive version. But it takes effort to do so. The first step is to simply become aware of and identify the voice. Many clients have said to me, "I wish I could just be nicer to myself." You can! It's your voice, after all, that's reflecting your feelings and fears back to you. You can choose to question your automatic thinking and replace hurtful statements with more rational, objective, and kind ones. My client, Joe, realized this when he decided to name his internal narrator "Larry." Why does Larry get a say about how Joe feels about himself? Why is Larry such an ass? What's his problem anyway? We'll get to the bottom of this awful story!

We're going to ignore the voice when it tells us that there must be something wrong with us or that we can never change. We'll keep going even when Squash says it's stupid or Larry calls us a loser, or we think we're wasting our time because this will never work and we're just not good enough. We're going to do it because deep down, we know better, and it's time for healthier voices to rise. It's your story. Don't you deserve a narrator who makes it a memorable and meaningful memoir?

It's time to *Fire Your Narrator!* if you:

- Constantly question yourself.

- Ruminate incessantly over past mistakes.

- Overthink situations to the point of inaction.

- Are your own worst critic.

- Hold yourself and others to impossible standards.

- Feel like nothing you do is good enough.

But wait, there's more!

Perhaps you're someone who:

- Is always worried about what other people think.

- Takes a small problem and makes it worse.

- Feels stuck and doesn't know what to do about it.

- Believes that nothing will ever change.

- Says things to yourself in your head that you'd never say to another person.

When that inner voice squashes your every move and moments of optimism, it's time to *Fire Your Narrator!* and cast a new voice.

If you can recast your narrator, you can reframe your past story. If you can reframe your past story, you can free yourself in the present to create a clearer, happier, and more satisfying future. The only thing you've got to lose is that unhelpful voice.

Squash what's squashing you. It's time to get out of your head and into your life.

## CHAPTER 1

# DON'T BELIEVE EVERYTHING YOU SAY

## *Everyone Is a Little Unreliable*

*"We are what we believe we are."* – C.S. Lewis

You're the type of person who gets things done. You're a helpful colleague, a trusted friend, and a good person. You're likely a high-achiever who seeks constant improvement. And because of that, you tend to be hard on yourself. You're convinced doing so will lead to a better version of you. You're focused on what you do for and how you interact with others. You haven't considered taking a look inside your own head.

Somewhere in the back of your mind is that voice that talks

to you throughout your day. It tends to remember bad things over good, negative experiences over positives, slights and embarrassments over accomplishments and pride. It focuses on your worst qualities, reminding you of things you'd prefer to forget. It keeps you up at night, ruminating on past mistakes. It makes you the center of every experience, even those that have nothing to do with you.

Externally, you look like you've got it all together.

Internally, you are a whirlwind of thoughts, emotions, doubts, and concerns.

The voice tells you that you don't measure up. It second-guesses your actions, often before you even have a chance to put them into action. It berates you for minor transgressions most wouldn't even notice, like that time you left your cellphone in the produce aisle by a pile of unripe avocados and spent the next 20 minutes running around the market in your flip-flops, totally freaking out. OK, that was me.

The voice questions the motives of others. They're only being nice because they're your friends. They don't want to hurt your feelings. Or they never measure up to your expectations and standards. They always let you down and cannot be trusted. You're clearly all alone! It sees things as absolutes and doesn't believe in the power of growth or change or experiences as lessons learned.

But why? Why would you choose to narrate your life this way?

Would you believe this voice thinks it is protecting you? It's triggered by fear and worries of inadequacy. It believes it's keeping you safe. It is a constant presence, a seemingly trusted companion that is entirely untrustworthy.

Your narrator is a uniquely internalized individual, a combination of early voices and stories you were told or came to believe about yourself. Over the years, you tended to disregard all evidence to the contrary, filtering out feedback that didn't support these internal beliefs.

The voice grew louder and more confident. It's been along for the ride, occasionally making you more productive but more often than not keeping you stuck, hypercritical of yourself and others, and ultimately unhappy.

If we're going to look for what's true, we've got to start with a hard truth:

You're a liar.

It's OK. Stay with me. I'm a liar too. We all are in some way.

You're also pretty unreliable.

That's OK too. So am I.

This doesn't mean you're not a good person or that you don't show up for others. I believe you are and that you do. You should believe this also. But let's get real. You've been lying to yourself for years. You shouldn't believe everything you tell yourself.

You fill your head with untruths, and then, because you've gained your own trust, you believe the things you believe. Even when they hurt. Even when they're unhelpful. Even when your best friend says, "Stop talking that way about my best friend!" because hearing you say it about yourself hurts her too. Why would you say such mean things to the person you should care for the most? I'm not talking about your mom, your spouse, your significant other, or even your dog. I'm talking about you. Who should care more about you than you?

You're unreliable because we all are, at least a little bit. Not because you forgot you signed up to provide napkins for the second-grade class party, and now all the students are going home with frosting in their hair (been there), or because you didn't make it home from your work trip in time to tuck your toddler into bed because you didn't hear them announce your delayed flight was ready to depart because you were too busy drinking in the airport bar (been there too).

But I digress.

If there's one thing you can rely on, it's that every narrator is at least a little unreliable.

In literature, the unreliable narrator is the character voicing the story, whose own take on that story is somewhat compromised. The reader has enough information to question the narrator's version of the story. That doesn't mean it's not a fun ride, experiencing the story through this lens, but it does make the reader somewhat skeptical of the *interpretation* of events. The narrator clearly has a point of view that isn't entirely or factually correct. We love following an unreliable narrator's narrative and rooting for them to learn, grow, and discover more about themselves in order for them to ultimately succeed.

Your narrator is unique in its unreliability. That's because our past experiences are processed through a particular lens, creating a powerful inner thinking. Because of our tendency to remember negative or harmful events far more than typical, uneventful ones, we hold on to those memories longer.[1] And then, we look to our past as evidence when contemplating our present. Meaning, if we're far more likely to remember or be fearful of a negative incident, we're always on the lookout for more of the same. We approach with caution and avoid the conflict at all costs.

Sometimes this holds us back. Often it allows us to reaffirm what we already know: bad things happen and thus must be avoided. That confirmation bias shows up in our behaviors, choices, actions and reactions. The bias solidifies in our narrative point of view – the way we view the world – and ultimately creates that inner narrator that serves as the voice-over of our daily lives.

When we're only looking to the past for evidence and we're seeing it through a compromised lens, we don't see the present opportunities to change the story. We continue with the same behaviors and actions that solidify our existing inner narrative into our external reality.

At work, the unreliable narrator might show up this way: On Friday, you turned in a strategic analysis to your boss, Danita. You felt a bit rushed on this project, and given your high standards, you don't feel 100% confident of your conclusions. Then again, you never do. You always think you could have done it better. This one feels particularly important because you've felt lately like you're walking on eggshells with Danita. Nothing you do seems to make

---

[1] This sucks, but it's true. Scientific studies show we're all hanging onto the negatives way more than the positives. https://www.ncbi.nlm.nih.gov/pmc/articles/PMC2676782/

her happy. She didn't even say thanks when you rushed to finish and give her the file before she left early for the weekend. Now it's Monday morning, and you pass her in the hallway. You say hi and give a friendly wave. And – she walks right past you without even acknowledging your presence.

"Oh no," you think. "It's my report. It's no good. She hates it."

Your stomach sinks.

Unreliable narrator? Quite possibly!

What evidence do you have that Danita didn't like your work? None, yet. Just a story, one created by fear, not facts. You don't think, "Gee, maybe Danita didn't hear me. Maybe Danita was late to a meeting and has her own busy agenda this morning. Maybe Danita ate some bad carbonara last night and had to run to the bathroom." You just don't know! Your inner narrator makes it about you, highlighting some flaw or concern, and makes a bigger story out of that single interaction.

No situation is ever exactly as it seems. There are intricacies, nuances, and interpretations. And yet, the inner narrator seeks to compartmentalize it all into a simple story. The brain seeks to confirm its beliefs. If you constantly tell yourself, "Things never work out for me," you'll notice all the times things don't work out and ignore the times they do.

Say you have an employee, Bill, who is habitually late. You explain the necessity of arriving at work on time. Four out of the next five days, Bill arrives on time, but on Friday he is again late. You're far more likely, as his boss who is already aware of this behavior, to notice Bill's one day of tardiness – confirming the conclusions you have already made ("Bill is always late! He clearly doesn't care about his work!") – rather than the two previous days when he arrived on time and the two days when he was actually in early. It's an uphill battle for Bill to change your mind.

The only thing that you can rely on is that your narrator will always be at least a little unreliable! Everyone's is. Our job is to question our narrative point of view and seek evidence of the truth. If we can question our beliefs, we can hold inner storylines up for review and reject the ones found to be false. We can stop Squash in her tracks and tell her to stand down. We can create a better story.

In the following chapters we'll explore 10 types of narrators that frequently appear. We'll learn how to recognize and combat them and how to rewrite them. The list is neither finite nor exhaustive but a representation of the statements I've heard from dozens of clients and hundreds of audience members. The unreliable narrator can be considered the overarching type, used from here on out as an umbrella term. Beneath that umbrella of unreliability are 10 narrator archetypes. See if you recognize your inner voice in the following descriptions. Some may seem more familiar than others. Several may overlap in your own experience.

We each have our own unique combination of these narrative types. As you read the following chapters, consider if the narrator description sounds like you and how frequently the sayings or thought process representative of that type show up. Note whether you tend to hear or think them (1) "Often" (daily), (2) "Sometimes" (occasionally, and especially when stressed), or (3) "Never" (unfamiliar). You likely have clear tendencies toward two or three narrative types with others as secondary characteristics. Through this exercise, you can map your own inner narrator and review the steps to correct and redirect the voice serving in this all-important role.

The 10 unreliable narrative types and their catchphrases include:

- The Critical Narrator: *You're Not Good Enough*

- The Runaway Narrator: *Where Are You Headed?*

- The Overthinking Narrator: *What's on Your Mind?*

- The Arrogant Narrator: *It's Not Me, It's You*

- The Self-Centered Narrator: *It Is Me, Isn't It?*

- The Ruminating Narrator: *Don't Forget (About This Awful Thing)*

- The Adamant Narrator: *That's Just the Way It Is (and Will Always Be)*

- The Defeatist Narrator: *What's the Point?*

- The People-Pleasing Narrator: *Love Me! Need Me! Want Me!*

- The Striving Narrator: *More Is Never Enough*

The following pages will allow you to identify, question, and address your inner narrator. Ultimately, your narrator is nothing more than a subjective point of view. Squash simply solidifies past stories in present situations and predicts a similar future. Your story can be rewritten. You can fire your narrator and cast a better one.

Read on.

CHAPTER 2

# THE CRITICAL NARRATOR

## *You're Not Good Enough*

Let's start with the most critical stuff, shall we? When most people think of an inner voice, they call it their inner critic. It's that voice that scolds, reprimands, criticizes, and belittles every effort. It's a voice deeply ingrained from childhood memories of being admonished by the teacher or rejected by our first love.

The Critical Narrator is constantly judging our behavior before and during a choice or action and most definitely after. It's why some people have called the inner critic our "personal bully" or our "inner asshole"[2] or the "madwoman in the attic."[3] It says things we'd never dream of saying to someone else but have no issue saying to ourselves.[4]

"I'm so stupid!" you might say after spilling coffee all over your desk. "I'll never get anything done," you insist, feeling overwhelmed at the lengthy project you've yet to start because you've been binging all six seasons of *Schitt's Creek* – for the second time.

"Ugh, look at you," you wail in the unflattering light of the dressing room. "Why would you think you can wear horizontal stripes?"

Can you imagine if we said such things to anyone else? We'd get punched in the face! Or, at a minimum, we'd find we don't get many social invites. Instead, we invite and allow those shots to our own face, and our psyche, by ourselves!

My friend Tanya knows me well enough to know my inner critic is always at work. "I know no matter what I say, you're still going to beat yourself up over this," she once said to me. (I can't actually remember what "this" was, but it must have seemed very important at the time.) "So, if you're going to beat yourself up anyway, use a feather and not a club."

---

[2] Jen Pastiloff hysterically refers to her narrator as her "inner asshole" in her beautifully written memoir, *On Being Human*, which you need to read ASAP!
[3] The "madwoman in the attic," a reference to Charlotte Brontë's *Jayne Eyre*, is how sisters Emily Nagoski, PhD, and Amelia Nagoski, DMA, refer to the inner voice in their 2019 book, *Burnout: The Secret to Unlocking the Stress Cycle*, which you should also read ASAP!
[4] Seriously, why are you still here? There are clearly better books to read.

Use a feather. Not a club. Genius.

Why be your own worst enemy? We have enough evil villains to fight in our story. Don't be one of them.

## Tips to Critique a Critical Narrator:

- Consider what you're saying to yourself. What's the point of the thought? Is it helpful? Or hurtful? How might you turn critical commentary into helpful advice?

- Allow for a compliment to complement every criticism. If you're going to pick apart something you did, give equal attention to what went right as well as what you would change or improve.

- Consider if a friend had made such a mistake or faced a similar dilemma. What might you say to her? Try talking to yourself as you would to your best friend. Share the same words of support with yourself.

- Respond to that critical inner voice with a simple question: "*So what?*" So what if you failed the test, blew the interview, or spilled the coffee? In the grand scheme of your life, what is the meaning of this one moment? This is only one part of the story, and a small one at that.

- Remind yourself that you've survived every mistake you've made up to this point. You'll survive this one too.

- Who made you head judge? Ask yourself why it's your job

to serve as judge and jury for everything you do and if your standards need to be so stringent. What does "winning" look like, anyway?

- Laugh a little. There's humor to be had – and relatable stories to share – as a result of your shortcomings. Own your missteps.

- If none of the above work, it's also OK to tell yourself to shut up. Maybe not out loud, because that would be weird, but definitely in your own head.

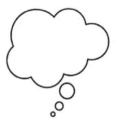

## CHAPTER 3

# THE RUNAWAY
# NARRATOR

## *Where Are You Headed?*

What's an unreliable narrator with a full tank of gas? A Runaway one. The Runaway Narrator takes the unreliable narrator on the fast track into the future without bothering to check if the destination is one worth visiting.

The Critical Narrator says of the boss's rebuff: "Danita didn't acknowledge me in the hall. She must have hated my project."

The Runaway Narrator then picks up the storyline and … runs with it. "I can't believe I screwed it up. I can't do anything right. I'm so going to get fired. What will I do if I get fired? It's a bad time to be out of work. The job market is tight, and I haven't updated my résumé in years. My life sucks. I'm going to be unemployed forever, and I have no friends and will die alone with no one by my side but my 12 cats."

You get the point.

What just happened here? It's like picking a train at the station without asking where it's going. We're not only forecasting what might happen next, we're on the express to doomsday.

The Runaway Narrator takes the story into a predetermined future. Although that's frequently a future of disappointment, dread, and dying among a dozen cats, the train can chug unchecked in the other direction too. It's why we should always look at the fine print on the ticket before jumping on board.

Consider "Cathy," who called me in excitement one day. Could I recommend a realtor to put their house on the market? Cathy had landed a coveted second interview for a role she really wanted. The company was flying her to Florida to meet with the team, so they certainly seemed interested. And living in Florida would be so great. She'd already researched the best schools for her kids. And they could get a pool – everyone in Florida has a pool! Look at this adorable unicorn float – wouldn't that look great in the pool? Cathy felt things were finally working out for her. It would all depend on how much they could get for their current house. They were eager to get it on the market, stat, and secure the sale.

Whoa, slow down there, Cathy! Cathy's Runaway Narrator has already gotten her the job, sold and bought property, and is happily sucking down mojitos on her unicorn float in her Florida pool. It's an appealing place to be, but she's already three chapters ahead in the story. We're not quite there yet!

I'm all for the power of positive thinking. I believe in visualizing an ideal future and taking action to get there. But in this case, a few things need to happen before Cathy does something as drastic as entertaining offers on her current home. Cathy's got to get the job. In fact, even before that, she has to nail the interview, so the potential employer will want to offer her the job. No great interview, no job offer. No job offer, no moving. Even if she gets the job, she has to make sure that the offer is sufficient and worthy of uprooting her family.

You want to envision your family in this new location? Great! Do some research. You want to know how much your house is worth should you need to put it on the market? Get a quote. Don't put it up for sale just yet, Cathy. You want an adorable unicorn float for your pool? Bookmark some websites, or start a Pinterest board, but don't shop online for pool toys for the new pool in the new home you haven't bought because *you don't yet have the job.*

An unfortunate but unsurprising follow-up: Cathy had a great interview. But she didn't get the job. She was, however, able to use the interest from other companies to leverage her status at work. She eventually got a promotion and is happier in her role and with her present company. And they still live in the same house, in the same school system, with plenty of money left over for an annual Florida vacation.

Before you jump on that train, don't get ahead of the story. Don't let a Runaway Narrator run off with your future without being solidly on board.

## Tips to Redirect a Runaway Narrator:

- Decide if this particular thought-train is a worthy ride. Stop at the station before securing a seat.

- Ground yourself in the present before heading into the future story. Plot points happen one at a time, and pivots and detours are likely. Accept that there is no one set outcome and that change is always possible.

- If your Runaway Narrator tends to head straight to doomsday, stop first and ask yourself why you're predicting the worst possible outcome. What might be an alternative "optimal outcome?" By visualizing the desired outcome, you can align your actions accordingly.

- Consider the "first, next step." You don't need to have every move perfectly choreographed to proceed.

- If what will truly make you happy is a unicorn float, give yourself permission to buy one.

# A STORY:
## This One's for You, Judgy McJudgeface

One time, when my kids were little, I was angry that laundry had been left in the dryer for what seemed like days, apparently awaiting the arrival of the Magic Cleaning Fairy to fold and put it all away. The laundry basket, which should have held piles of neatly folded clothes, sat empty atop the dryer. This infuriated me so much, I summoned my inner Carli Lloyd taking a penalty shot on goal.

In a huff, I kicked the empty laundry basket down the hallway while loudly declaring (aka shouting): "WHY AM I THE ONLY ONE WHO DOES ANYTHING AROUND HERE?"

A few days later, I sent my young son to his room to pick up his toys. He was mad, and instead of picking up his toys, he proceeded to kick them across the room while yelling, "WHY AM I THE ONLY ONE WHO DOES ANYTHING AROUND HERE?"

Oopsie.

What is it they say? Imitation is the most sincere form of flattery?

Not my finest moment.

Among dozens of other "not-so-fine" moments.

I mess up. A lot.

And then, as if to make up for all my mess-ups, I berate myself incessantly thereafter.

For years after.

The "laundry basket incident" was nearly a decade ago. My kids have no memory of it.

But I can't forget and continue to judge myself years later. Here's when Squash shows up to squash my best efforts and remind me that I'm a bad mom, an impatient mom, a mom who yells.

Here's what Squash insists: A better mom would handle that situation calmly and with ease.

Here's how far Squash will run with that narrative: A better mom enjoys the task of folding laundry and spritzing it with lavender essential oil before carefully adding perfectly folded shirts and undies to the organized drawers of the appropriate dressers. And she'll do so with a smile.

I'm not that mom.

And because I know I'll never measure up to that mom, Squash puts me on trial for that transgression and others just as small.

How small?

I'm the mom who was miffed when someone else signed up to provide plates and napkins for the class party. That's my domain, where my name always goes. Clearly, I'm selfish and possessive, and I DON'T BAKE!

I'm the mom who sent her kindergartner to school on the day there was no kindergarten and sheepishly returned to the principal's office later to retrieve him after getting a call at work saying that I clearly don't love my kids enough to pay attention to the ever-rotating winter advisory, half-day kindergarten schedule. Or, at least, that's what I imagined they said.

So that must mean I'm forgetful and disorganized, and WHAT DAY OF THE WEEK IS IT AGAIN?

I dislike when the home phone rings late at night, at dinnertime, or really any time. I hate having to call any service provider that requires me to deal with an automated response line. I'm the irate customer who immediately and angrily presses every button, shouting, "REPRESENTATIVE!"

Because I'm impatient and easily frustrated, and WHY CAN'T A HUMAN BEING PICK UP THE PHONE?

You know those glass half-full and glass half-empty people?

I'm neither. I can't find my glass. WHERE DID I LEAVE MY GLASS?

That's me, yelling at myself in my head. Sometimes I yell out loud to let the volume out. Parenting books will tell you this is one of the worst things you can do to your kids. And don't ever do this while watching your kids play sports. You're not supposed to yell or cheer. They now have "silent sidelines," and you're only allowed to mime clap for every player on each team and then to tell your kids later, in the sincerest way, that you just love to watch them play. And no, you're not going to get a post-game snack from the Good Humor man because — added fructose and corn syrup. But take these homemade gluten-free granola bars I so carefully cut into individual serving sizes and wrapped in nontoxic, biodegradable packaging so you can give one to every one of your food-intolerant teammates.

I once had a mug that declared me "World's Greatest Mom." I don't have that mug anymore. I don't know where it is. Maybe someone found out about me and took it away.

With Squash in my ear, I'd rate myself a four and a half out of 10.

I'm a very judgmental Judge Judy.

And who I judge most harshly is myself.

I get upset at little things, like when the power goes out for a blip and all of the clocks in the house need to be reset. Why are there so many digital clocks in this house? How does one get them to display the same time?

Sometimes I get a productive rush, and I tend to multiple tasks at once.

I feel powerful, like I can accomplish anything!

Then I arrive in a room and can't recall why I am there.

I wait for a minute, hoping it will come back to me.

Nope, it's gone.

Never mind.

I never balance the checkbook, can't help my kids with algebra, and need someone else to figure out how to split the bill.

I forget every password I have. I keep resetting the passwords and then forgetting them again. Why is this so hard?

I'm disorganized and fretful! And let's not forget lazy and a little lumpy too.

Like the Russian judge who takes points off for minor infractions, I can't give myself a break. I'm Judge Judgeanova. It doesn't matter how difficult the daily routine was to complete if I didn't stick the landing with a smile.

If you're a judgy type, too, you waste your days criticizing your best efforts, focusing on your failures, and passing off successes to someone else.

Here's what I can tell you, Judgy McJudgeface, from one judge to another. There's no one scoring this thing but us.

There's no podium or gold medal or victory photo on a Wheaties box.

There is, most likely, an empty Wheaties box in my pantry because someone finished the box but neglected to take it out with the recycling.

And that's because, clearly, I'M THE ONLY ONE WHO DOES ANYTHING AROUND HERE.

# CHAPTER 4

# THE OVERTHINKING NARRATOR

## *What's on Your Mind?*

An Overthinking Narrator is overstressed. It's always on. Always thinking, questioning, analyzing, and positioning without ever being able to just *be* and let things happen. The Overthinking Narrator loves information. Bits and pieces of it. In fact, it can't proceed until it has *all* the information. And, of course, you can never have all the information.

If you feel like you just can't shut off your brain and you need to know every possible option or every potential outcome before you can make a decision, you might have an Overthinking Narrator. The Overthinker delays our decision-making and causes consternation and distress while overanalyzing all options. At worst, it keeps us stuck for weeks, months, even years, with decisions, many of which aren't worth the time spent debating them.

Molly's husband is an Overthinker. He's always seeking to sort and process information before deciding. On anything. This drives her nuts. It took him months to buy sunglasses, she tells me. He wanted to make sure he was getting the frame and type that looked best and at the best price. Throw in a warranty and a few shipping options and the process would take at least another week. Why does this bother Molly? She points out while she appreciates his attention to detail and price-conscious purchasing habits, they sometimes miss out on opportunities because of the delay. Like waiting for airline ticket prices to drop and finding they triple instead. No trip for Molly. At the mall, he'll insist they can find a desired item less expensive elsewhere, only to find it sold out everywhere a week later. No item for Molly.

This sets her off. Just buy the darn thing! And his response, thinking through all the possibilities, is that Molly's not thinking it through enough. He finds her decision-making rash and often faulty, one that doesn't ultimately maximize their investment.

On the plus side, Molly points out, once her husband makes a decision, based on the amount of time he's spent deliberating it, he sticks with it. I asked about the sunglasses that took months to buy. He loves them. The car she'd like for him to upgrade is going strong after 11 years. She says he has a bathrobe as old as their relationship. And they've been married for 20 years. He loves that bathrobe. She admits if he can hold onto a bathrobe that long, despite its wear and shabbiness, it bodes well for her, his wife, and her stretched and weathered future. She smiles when she tells me about the bathrobe.

She momentarily stops overthinking their relationship.

Does your Overthinking Narrator ask a lot of questions? The Overthinking Narrator's twin sister is the Overquestioner. It's always investigating for the hidden story and wondering what else is at play. Will this work? What's a better option? Why did that happen? What should I do now?

Here's where the Overthinker meets the Runaway Narrator. Let's say a friend cancels lunch plans. Maybe the timing wasn't good for her. Maybe she got busy. Or maybe it's something else. The Overthinker might think: "Does it mean she doesn't want to be my friend anymore? Did I do something to upset her? Was it because I told her the tile backsplash she chose for her kitchen was a bit 'bold'? Should I text her? Or maybe call her? Or stop by with flowers?"

Overthinking and Overquestioning Narrators lack a trust in themselves that's necessary to make decisions and stand by them. They become so accustomed to questioning their choices that every choice becomes one of analysis and decision delay. Clients of mine say they wish they could turn down the volume on those questioning thoughts and worry less about the "what if?"

The good news is, they can. It starts, surprisingly, by questioning the thoughts themselves and thinking (but not *overthinking*) about better ones.

## Tips to Outmatch the Overthinking Narrator:

- Acknowledge you'll never have all the answers. How much information do you truly need to make a decision? Consider that in most scenarios, there's no one right answer. Proceed with what seems like the best option.

- For actions that require research, keep your need for knowledge to a time-specific deadline appropriate to the urgency and importance of the task. (I'll spend 20 minutes looking at boots on Zappos and then just select a pair to try on – after all, they have free returns, and I can always order another!)

- Consider your need for control. Even with all the information, you can't always control the outcome or direct every scene. Learn to manage your emotional response to the situation rather than the situation itself.

- Not all decisions require the same amount of information. Practice those decision-making skills with choices that aren't of huge consequence. Omelet or French toast? Both sound great. Which should you get? You can't really go wrong here. If you're so disappointed when your eggs arrive that it's going to ruin your day, you can always order a pancake on the side.

- Why fear the consequences? There's always another choice to make. You make a wrong choice; you get to make a new one. We have an endless supply of choices. The only choice that removes our agency is when we think we have no choice.

- Action is the antidote to anxiety. To maintain forward momentum, take small steps out of your thinking and questioning mind and put action into play. You'll move the story forward and get some answers to your endless questions.

- You want the true test of overcoming your overthinking? Try not to overthink these tips.

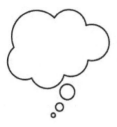

# CHAPTER 5

# THE ARROGANT NARRATOR

## *It's Not Me, It's You*

It's uncomfortable to admit this, but I can be a bit arrogant. I'm not totally self-absorbed, admiring my reflection in the mirror all day (I tend to avoid mirrors unless the lighting is quite good and I've had a professional makeover first), but I do tend to think I'm right. Not all the time, of course. But … a lot of the time.

Call it a healthy ego. I have enough evidence to know that I work hard, generally make sane decisions, and won't let someone down. If you give me something to do, I will get it done and for the most part, unless it's like complicated macramé or advanced physics, I can do it well. I'm also OK admitting when I'm wrong, which is the right thing to do and consequently also makes me right, even when I'm wrong.

I wasn't always like this. I was a shy kid who worried incessantly. My teens and 20s were full of insecurities. My 30s were a blur, trying to manage family and work while suffering from imposter syndrome and feeling like I was always letting someone down. My 40s became about reinvention. I was tired of trying to be everything to everyone and decided for the first time in a long time to put myself at the top of my own list. A healthy assertiveness was born. I no longer see myself as the problem in every situation. I see room for opportunity and growth without berating myself for my shortcomings. I've learned to quiet Squash. It took a long time, but I feel like I've finally arrived at a place where I can take ownership of me. There's a lot that's right about me, and I don't think it's wrong to acknowledge that.

An assertive narrator is a confident narrator. Assertiveness becomes arrogance when no one else can meet my own personal expectations. Did no one prepare for today's meeting? Why am I the only one who takes these meetings seriously? It's like no one else does anything around here or even cares. And at home – what's with the dishwasher? Can't all you people who live in this house see that it's full and set it to run? And once it's done, why can't the kids put the clean dishes away in the cabinets, where they belong? Why do they always wait for me to do it? And when they do it, they put the dishes back in the wrong places. And I have to redo it. How many times do I have to tell them to divide up the salad forks from the dinner forks? Don't just stick them in the same place – that's why we have a divided cutlery draw holder thingy that I bought for $19.99 at Bed, Bath & Beyond. It's impossible to keep things organized when the rest of you keep messing it all up. That's just wrong.

You get where I'm going with this, right? The Arrogant Narrator says I'm right and you're wrong, and that's probably why nobody wants to put the dishes away – because they know I'm going to get irritated with them for not doing it to my standards. There is a right way to do things, and it is *my* way. Me, me, me. All for me. Mine.

Does this sound harsh? You should know I don't save this type of judgment for my family alone. I judge strangers too. Like when I'm in a long line at Subway to get a sandwich and the person in front of me gets to the counter and they don't know what they want. You're only now just looking at the menu? You had all this time to figure out what you wanted while waiting in line, and just now, you realized you have to think about what you're actually going to order? Seriously, it's Subway, how hard can this be? If you're not ready, how about I go ahead of you since I'm the only one here who knows how to order a sandwich?

If any of this sounds remotely familiar to you, rest assured you're not alone. Having an Arrogant Narrator is not necessarily a negative thing. Sure, you can be a little rigid and impatient, but you've got a healthy self-confidence that can be channeled to work with you and not against others. An Arrogant Narrator doesn't make you a bad person. Being aware of your tendency to think you're (always) right is the first step. Understanding that everybody has their own internal story and that yours isn't the only or right one is the second. And that there might be more than one way to correctly unload the dishwasher. Maybe.

## Tips to Adjust an Arrogant Narrator:

- Admit that there's more than one way to do things. Be open to learning and discovery. There's nothing wrong with being wrong. There may be repercussions to thinking you are always right.

- Recognize people's contributions and skills in areas other than your own. Everyone brings value, even if their contributions aren't always immediately apparent.

- Decide what's worth speaking up about and what you can let go. Do you always need to be the one to notice and fix everything? What would happen if you stopped doing that? If you step back occasionally, you might find others willing to step up.

- Allow yourself to be human and to be accepting of other humans. No one is good at everything. Flaws are endearing. Practice compassion and forgiveness – with yourself and for others.

- Consider that there are worse things in the world than having the dinner and salad forks mixed together in the utensil divider.

## CHAPTER 6

# THE SELF-CENTERED NARRATOR

## *It* Is *Me,* Isn't It?

The Self-Centered Narrator is the Arrogant Narrator's less-confident second cousin, once removed. The Self-Centered Narrator has a way of making every story about itself but not because it wants to be the center of the story. It just thinks it is.

Say you walk into a room, and suddenly, people start whispering. You feel self-conscious. What are they saying? Are they whispering about you? Did you do something silly? Do you have a "kick me" sign on your shirt? Or your boss is griping about how far behind the team is on a current project. You're not the lead of the project, but you take it as a reprimand about your own performance. Or you meet up with friends, and when you arrive, they're all laughing.

You ask what's so funny, and they brush it off. "Never mind," they say. "You wouldn't get it."

Do you automatically assume each of these situations is about you? You might suffer from a Self-Centered Narrator. The Self-Centered Narrator always puts herself in the middle of the action and personalizes the situation. She's sensitive to feedback from others, no matter how small. She's in tune with tiny slights but often out of touch with the real story. Got a molehill? She'll make it a mountain. It's always about her and her story.

You probably know someone like this whose daily dramas steal the spotlight. Yet in your own life, you don't want the spotlight shining too brightly on you, unless you can know for sure you'll look and sound good and glow with confidence. You'd like attention – but only when you can fully control the scene.

Having that type of Self-Centered Narrator can make you socially self-conscious and leads to perfectionism and anxiety. It's strongly aligned with the Critical Narrator, always judging performance and assuming that an internal flaw is responsible for external situations. It's the difference between saying, "I need to fix this situation," and "this situation needs fixing."

It's not selfish to want to calm a Self-Centered Narrator. It's a matter of survival.

## Tips to Soothe a Self-Centered Narrator:

- Recognize it's not always about you. You are the center of *your* world but not everyone else's. They're mostly worried about themselves, just as you're worried about yourself.

- Get perspective. Ask someone you trust for their take on a situation that's causing you distress or that you may be overanalyzing.

- Get clarification. Want better answers? Ask more specific questions. To your boss: "Is there anything I could be doing better or more of to assist you and the team?"

- Presume positive intent. Admit to your close friend: "When you all laughed when I arrived, I thought I might be the butt of the joke." You'll get the real story and then can decide how to feel about the information you've received.

- Understand that every situation is a unique combination of characters and plot points. No one person is responsible for everything and everyone. A pitcher may give up the game-winning run in the bottom of the ninth, but the rest of the team played a role in getting them to that game-defining moment.

- Don't be afraid to speak up and seek out attention for the right reasons. Be positive, be generous, and be willing to make a mistake or even fail. In short, be human. (You know you're allowed to be human, right?)

# CHAPTER 7

# THE RUMINATING NARRATOR

## *Don't Forget (About This Awful Thing)*

The Ruminating Narrator loves to remember things. In particular, it remembers not very good things, holding on to and replaying unfortunate memories more frequently than they deserve to be remembered. And because of our propensity to recall negative experiences more vividly and frequently than positive ones,[5] the Ruminating Narrator spends more time replaying bad experiences from our past, which only serves to make us feel worse in the present.

We often ruminate on situations of little consequence that

---

[5] Remember, this isn't just Squash talking. It's science. See Chapter 1.

others have long forgotten:

The admonishment from your boss when you sent an email intended for one person to the entire department.

That time you slipped in the cafeteria in fifth grade and went down hard in front of Luke, that boy you liked but thought would never notice you. He did, on that day, as you lay on the floor with a tray of Tater Tots scattered on your torso.

Or that time you led the morning meeting and expectorated on a platter of pastries. That means spit on, for those of you unfamiliar with the polite descriptive. What? You've never spit on a platter of pastries? Oh, right, that was me, again. It's the stuff that keeps me up at night, but it's kind of a funny story.

Read on...

# A STORY:
# What Do You Do When You Accidentally Spit on a Donut?

I wake up at 2:30 a.m. with a thought.

It's not about all I have to do when my alarm goes off in just three hours (though I often do think about that). It's not about whether I left the stove on or the garage door open (though I sometimes obsess about that too).

It's not even about the tabby cat lying on my stomach and kneading my bladder with her paws and whether I should get up before I accidentally pee in my bed (thankful to say that hasn't actually happened … yet).

No, it's about something that happened some years ago. A contribution I made during a business breakfast meeting.

The fact that it was a breakfast meeting plays into the story because there were platters of pastries on the table. This I remember because I really wanted a croissant but didn't want to be the only one to reach for one and was thinking I'd just grab it on my way out the door when the meeting was done.

Anyway, I digress. (Pastries have that effect on me.) It's 2:30 in the morning, and I'm suddenly awake and thinking about what happened when I started speaking at this break-fast meeting.

All was going well until, along with my persuasive and impactful words, a tiny bit of spittle escaped from my mouth. I could see it fly through the air – minuscule though it was – and watched it land smack dab in the middle of the tray of pastries. Next to the croissant I was eyeing. Just to the left of the cranberry scone. On top of what I'm sure was, until that moment, a coveted chocolate donut.

And I froze for a second, unsure of protocol.

Had anyone else seen it? It was tiny. Please tell me no one else just saw that.

Should I apologize for unintentionally spitting on the tray of pastries? Should I pretend it didn't happen? Should I remove the now offensive item with a napkin?

Mortified, I continued, hoping no one would notice I just emitted bodily fluid and was turning as red as the center of a cherry danish.

What I had to say was important and effective. And I had ruined it by speaking so quickly and with such passion that I had somehow become unable to control my saliva and had accidentally Spit. On. A. Donut.

Yikes.

And here I am, at 2:30 in the morning, not the next day but some *three and a half years* later, revisiting that moment in all its horrifying detail.

To what purpose?

Now I'm wide awake and embarrassed, as if it has just happened, breaking into a sweat under the covers and feeling that shame and anger at myself all over again.

So why? Why now?

Why do memories, particularly unpleasant or unhelpful ones, continue to occupy our thoughts? And how do we stop them?

I'm a ruminator. Always have been. This story is just one example of the endless loop of gaffes, wrong moves, mistakes, and "constructive feedback" running on a tape through my head, often at the most inopportune times.

Like when I should be sleeping.

Or when I should be just moving on in my story rather than rereading a past and unpleasant chapter.

It's like I can't get past it.

For those unfamiliar, rumination is the "focused attention on the symptoms of distress and unpleasantness and on the consequences of negative actions or memories."

It's repetitively going over a thought or a problem without completion or without a solution.

An alternative definition of rumination has to do with cows.

Yes, cows.

Like chewing the cud – chewing again what has been chewed slightly and swallowed. It keeps coming back up and stays in your mouth (or brain) far longer than it should, a pasty, mealy meal.

Moo.

So, why do we do it? (Can I say "we" here? It can't be just me who does this, right? Let me ruminate on that.) What do we get from ruminating?

There's some belief – or relief – that if we continue to play the scene out in our minds, we may get it right.

The only way to do that is to rewrite it.

Ask yourself, "What's the meaning of this story? What value does it hold for me today? What's the benefit of continuing to revisit it in a way that brings me embarrassment or distress?"

You can't change the past – all the times you've disappointed yourself or fallen short or spit on a donut (really, how many times could you possibly have spit on a donut?) – so why are you replaying this past story and assigning it value in the present?

The stories we tell ourselves represent what's important to us. For me, that would be feeling foolish or making a mistake in front of people I want to impress, such as making an important and valuable point at a meeting only to worry the message was lost because, you know … that whole spitting on the donut thing. Understanding the root cause of the rumination – the feeling of failure or regret – is the first step in rewriting it.

Consider the difference between rumination and reflection. Reflection is an important process of looking back on our behavior and our actions and deciding if they truly represent who we want to be and how we want to behave. Reflection allows us to give serious thought or consideration to something from the past before moving on from it and creating room for growth and development. Rumination offers no such value. Rumination keeps us looped in regret. Break the habit of ruminating by actively acknowledging the loop of a story playing out in your mind. Habits are hard to break. Evaluate the objective facts of the event rather than your subjective narrative. You get to decide what meaning the event has for you. Stop assigning it more than it deserves.

Finally, laugh about it, at least a little.

Acclaimed novelist and screenwriter Nora Ephron said, "When you slip on a banana peel, people laugh at you. But when you tell people you slipped on a banana peel, it's your laugh."

I didn't slip on a banana peel. I spit on a donut. It had the unintended effect of getting me off my pastry habit. And when you think about it, it's kind of funny.

Maybe if I replace the meaning of that event, I can remember it with less embarrassment and with more amusement. We all have stories to tell. Stop ruminating on the regrettable ones.

## Tips to Rest a Ruminating Narrator:

- Rumination stems from unresolved issues. Create space and time to consider *why* you continue to stew in this thought. What's at the heart of the matter? If you struggle to do this on your own, seek a professional for additional support.

- Admit there's little benefit in replaying an embarrassing or disappointing scenario over and over again, particularly if it brings up unwanted emotions. Rather than reimagining the scene, *rewrite* it. Create in your head or your journal an alternative ending, one that feels satisfying and complete.

- Acknowledge that regret is a normal part of life. Use regret not as a method for reviewing the past but as a map for moving forward.

- Remember that past mistakes are present lessons learned and become great stories. Own your part in your own story, and turn the page to the next chapter.

- Don't underestimate the power of humor as a coping technique. Learn to laugh at yourself, and let others laugh along with you. (Donut, anyone?)

## CHAPTER 8

# THE ADAMANT NARRATOR

## *That's Just the Way It Is (and Will Always Be)*

The Adamant Narrator sees things clearly. Very clearly. Incredibly, awesomely, exceptionally clearly. Things are very black and white in the Adamant's world. There are no shades of gray. Not even the sort-of-sexy kind if you're into that type of thing.

When things are great – which they aren't that often – they are really, really great. And they never need to change. No need for growth when things are already pretty darn perfect.

When things are bad – which they are quite a bit more frequently – they are really, really bad. Terrible, really. And, what's worse, they will never change. Nope. The Adamant Narrator is adamant that how things are is how they will always be.

And when there's no middle ground, there can be no compromise. I once worked for an Adamant. He either loved you or hated you. There was no one he was lukewarm about. Unfortunately for me, I was one of the ones he hated. No matter what I did, he never saw the good in it. His feedback was always given in absolutes. "You're doing a terrible job," he'd inform me when there were a few mistakes in the show. "No one respects you," he'd let me know when an employee questioned me. And although I knew this wasn't entirely true, it still hurt. Rather than battle him, producing evidence to the contrary, I tried to invoke his help. "What can I do to improve?" I'd ask. He'd shake his head. "It is what it is," he informed me. "And that's all it will ever be."

Needless to say, I left that job shortly thereafter. There was little reason to prove myself when he wasn't looking for proof. He was adamant, and he was right, and nothing would change. Why bother to prove otherwise?

You may know someone like this. You may be like this. "No, I'm not!" you reply (adamantly, I might add). Consider the ways you hold your thoughts as irrevocable truths. You believe certain things about yourself, your relationships, and the situations you find yourself in. There is one way of looking at them. When things are good, you're reluctant to look at ways you can make them even better or to consider how others' experiences might not mirror your own.

But it's even more challenging when things are bad. When Adamant Narrators don't like where they are, they get stuck. They are stubborn and strong-willed and can become martyrs to their commitment to remaining so. To be wrong would be wrong so, they prove themselves right by staying exactly where they are.

Not so terrible if you're content where you are. But awful if you are not. Adamant Narrators are so certain they are right that they are oblivious to evidence that suggests otherwise. They'd rather sacrifice relationships, even sacrifice their own happiness, in their pursuit of the absolute certainty of their thought.

What's so good about being right if you're unhappy? What's so wrong about being wrong if you can change it? The first step for an Adamant Narrator is to acknowledge things won't always be as they are and to envision circumstances in a slightly different way. Be curious as to what may exist outside of your own adamant mind.

## Tips to Adjust an Adamant Narrator:

- Be aware of the Adamant's favorite words: *always* and *never*. Seek the ample space between those two extremes.

- Accept that situations and relationships are subject to change. Life is in a constant state of flux. There is no one predetermined destiny. Everything we choose to do has the potential to affect our future.

- Identify times when change led to better outcomes. Have you always had the same job, the same house, or the same relationship? What about the same dog or same wardrobe? (With the exception of Molly's husband's 20-year-old bathrobe, our clothing does tend to evolve.) What happened when those things changed?

- Acknowledge the journey. You weren't always where you are now. Where you'll be two weeks or two years or two decades from now may be an entirely different place.

- Do a cost-benefit analysis. What are the costs and the benefits of staying the same? What are the costs and benefits of change?

- Start with small changes. What might you try differently to get out of your own way? Like taking a different route to work or switching your purse to your other shoulder, you can retrain your brain to both do and think differently.

- Practice flexibility, literally. Stretch your body. Stretch your mind. Reach for new thoughts.

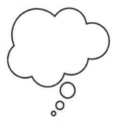

## CHAPTER 9

# THE DEFEATIST NARRATOR

## *What's the Point?*

The Defeatist Narrator is the sad sibling of the Adamant Narrator. It, too, believes things will never change, but the belief is built less on stubbornness and more on a debilitating case of pessimism.

The Defeatist is done before getting started. Like Eeyore, a Defeatist walks around with a giant cloud overhead. It's sunny elsewhere and raining only here! If you're a Defeatist, you have a hard time seeing the bright side of things or the potential for a better outcome. The Adamant says nothing will ever change, so I'm going to stay right where I am and do nothing, so there! The Defeatist says nothing's ever going to change, so why even bother trying? If the Defeatist Narrator had a musical accompaniment, it would be the world's tiniest violin. If it had a corresponding sound effect, it would be *womp womp*.

You poor little Defeatist Narrator! You're so run down, confused, and full of self-loathing that you've given up. What's the point in trying if you think nothing will change? Even worse, why hang around with optimists when they clearly don't understand your unfortunate circumstances? You'd rather decline the umbrella and stay in the rain. You won't look out at the horizon to see how the distant clouds are parting and will eventually reveal blue skies above. The Defeatist doesn't see the point – another rain cloud is sure to be close behind.

When the Defeatist Narrator stems from a larger issue, such as an underlying blanket of depression, a larger rewrite is necessary, and the cast of supporting characters needs to include professional resources. Reframing your narrator is part of the work to change the storyline.

## Tips to Defeat a Defeatist Narrator:

- Evaluate your situation. Are you suffering from something more than a Defeatist Narrator? Enlist the help of a licensed therapist, someone who can assess the severity and challenges of the situation.

- Identify times in the past in which your hard work paid off. Don't discount small successes. Did you learn a new recipe or finish a jigsaw puzzle? Tangible results serve as evidence.

- Focus on small activities that can help you feel a sense of positivity and momentum. Break bigger tasks into smaller ones. Want to earn a degree, but it all feels too overwhelming? Start by researching programs and seeing if you need to take a standardized test for admission. Before you can lose 50 lbs., you'll lose five.

- Surround yourself with optimistic people. Pessimism feeds on itself. Let someone else shine a light.

- Get some healthy perspective. Acknowledge all that's going right in your life. If you have clean running water, an ample food supply, and electricity, you're doing better than a third of the world's population. Volunteer. Read. Get out of your own head.

- Take care of your physical self. Get enough rest, sunlight, healthy nutrition, quiet time, and opportunities for fun. Small steps can lead to big changes. Start by believing that change is possible.

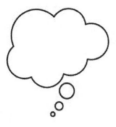

# CHAPTER 10

# THE PEOPLE-PLEASING NARRATOR:

## *Love Me! Need Me! Want Me!*

Whereas the Arrogant Narrator thinks it's all about them, the People-Pleasing Narrator thinks it's all about everybody else. What could be more noble than a life of service? If you're a People Pleaser, you're last on your list, if you even make it onto the list at all. Your energy goes elsewhere, helping others get what they need and where they want to go, with little saved for what you need to get to where you want to go. The People Pleaser hasn't thought about that at all.

The People-Pleasing Narrator wants you to drop everything to save your boss from the end-of-the-week fire drill that could have been avoided. You give your kids seconds of dessert, even though you haven't yet had a bite of yours. Your coffee gets cold while you make sure everyone else has a hot beverage. Of their choosing. In their favorite mug, even if it's the one you've been using. You'll just rinse it out. You weren't in the mood for that beverage anyway. It's all OK!

Oftentimes, the People-Pleasing Narrator will wind up feeling un- or underappreciated and taken for granted. Even resentful. You've martyred yourself for people who don't even care! But are the people you're so readily giving to actually asking for assistance? Could you assist the neighbor with picking up the mail once, but not as a daily task?

Raised to be polite, undemanding, and to put everyone else's needs before her own, the People Pleaser feels totally selfish saying no. You hate to let anyone down. Yet you'll let yourself down time and time again because you don't see your own worthiness.

"Kristal" came to me after years in marketing, wondering what's next in her career. She served as a "catchall" at work and was always rushing around. She was suffering from burnout. Given her years of experience and wealth of knowledge, colleagues relied on her to step in, solve problems, and salvage relationships. She became the go-to person for all sorts of tasks, including those outside the scope of her role and even outside of her department. Need something? Call Kristal; she'll know the answer, and she'll get it done! This went on for years. Despite feeling pulled in so many directions, she liked feeling needed and knowing she was contributing.

What do you get when you're the go-to person for all sorts of work? More work! Soon Kristal was inundated with tasks and projects that took up most of her time but offered little value to her own career. Jumping in to help others took away the time Kristal needed to focus on her own future. She lacked the time – any time – to truly think about what she wanted. She came to me for help in figuring out the next chapter in her life. Perhaps you feel the same – stuck where you are but too busy to even give thought to what comes next.

Planning a satisfying future starts with the simple step of taking the time to ask yourself, "What do *I* want?" Kristal didn't know. How could she when she has no time to think? She was frustrated by never being in control of her calendar and always working for someone else's benefit. We agreed that what she wanted most – right now – was time to think about what comes next. She started by blocking out an hour or two a week on her calendar reserved for "Kristal time." However she wanted to spend the time was entirely up to her.

What might that time look like? How about white space to reflect on which roles and tasks have been most satisfying? An opportunity to create a "brag book" of accomplishments to remind herself of her awesomeness? An hour to go to an exercise class, garden, or take a walk? Also appropriate. The only rule for Kristal was that she couldn't spend that time doing something for someone else. It was uncomfortable at first, but Kristal learned not only how to get back in touch with herself and her needs and wants, which ultimately helped her figure out her next career steps, but also that those other people in her life, from her boss to her husband, wouldn't fall apart without her for those 60 minutes.

Like Kristal, can you put yourself on your own list of people to please? What do you need to feel complete? What time might you carve out for yourself if others were taught to be less dependent on you? You matter. For as much as you care about other people's needs, consider your own. And then make them matter.

## Tips to Pacify a People-Pleasing Narrator:

- Allow yourself to be human. Like others in your story, you're entitled to your own wants, needs, and desires. Don't be so busy taking care of others that you neglect your own needs.

- Many people pleasers get pleasure from serving others, and there's no need to stop cold turkey. Learn to set boundaries, starting small. Say "no" to something you truly don't want to do. It might have little impact on the asker and a lot of impact for you.

- Block out time on your calendar for yourself. This time is sacred, so don't use it as a catchall. Be intentional with how you plan for this time. How might you spend it in a way that's just for you?

- Get comfortable with give and take. Don't enable someone else's dependence on you. Remind your inner narrator that your job is also to take care of yourself and that you'll be doing a favor to others by allowing them the opportunity to become self-sufficient.

- Get over the idea that everybody needs you to take care of their needs all of the time. Most people can figure things out on their own without you coming to the rescue.

- What do you want? No, really – take a minute to think about it. What do *you* want? If you've spent so long taking care of everyone else that you've lost sight of who you are, take some time to get to know yourself again. Create a likes and dislikes list. Revisit old hobbies and consider new ones. Meet yourself again, where you are now.

# A STORY:
## Stop Running for Someone Else's Hot Dog

This is a story about a hot dog.

But, really, it's about more than a hot dog.

The hot dog story takes place at a ballgame. We had nose-bleed-high seats near the top of the stadium. Many stairs up. Two innings in, a large family arrived to fill the rest of our row.

We stood to let them pass to their seats.

As soon as they got settled, the mom offered to get food for the family. (How did I know she was the mom? Maybe it was all those kids yelling, "MOM!" in her direction.)

She headed out (we stood to let her pass), down the many stairs.

She came back in the bottom of the third – lines were long at concessions – climbing the stairs cautiously with cardboard containers precariously stacked. We stood to let her pass, and she handed out the various hot dogs to each recipient.

But one was without its requested ketchup.

Oops!

And she was short on napkins.

Oh no!

Worst of all, she realized she had completely forgotten to take her husband's order. He had no hot dog!

Sucks for you, Dad!

She immediately offered to go back for the missing items, and moments later, arms now unloaded, off she went (we stood to let her pass, yup, again), down the stairs.

(Here's where I'm thinking Hubby can get his own damn hot dog.)

The lines must have still been crazy long because she didn't make it back up the stairs until the bottom of the fourth (we stood to let her pass) when she handed out the remaining food.

About two minutes later, one of the kids needed to go to the bathroom.

Of course.

So off she went again (we stood to let her pass), down the stairs with junior in tow.

Back they came, quads again activated up the stairs – at the top of the fifth. (We stood to let her pass – kind of the theme for the day.)

That was about the time her family started asking for dessert – several ice-cream sundaes in those plastic helmet cups, one cotton candy.

We resisted the urge (as we stood to let her pass) to place our own order as well. I mean, if she's going to keep going up and down these stairs, how hard would it be to bring back a few bottles of water?

I'll cut the story short here to recap:

This woman came to a baseball game but missed nearly all of it because she was so busy running errands for her family – back and forth, up and down the stairs, orders and reorders, bathroom breaks, and baseball helmet sundaes.

I want to be clear I was not judging. I was simply observing.

I don't know her story.

Maybe she hates baseball and had no interest in the game. Maybe she lives to serve. Maybe it's absolutely none of my business.

But it got me thinking, not about her story but about mine.

And yours.

And everyone's.

What's your hot dog?

Huh?

Your symbolic hot dog, silly.

I'll put it in quotes so you get the symbolism. What is the "hot dog" in your life that you keep running for, up and down the stairs, to serve to someone else?

How often do you put the needs of your "family" ahead of your own? (And your "family" can mean your work colleagues, your dramatic friend, the angry lady ahead of you in line in CVS, etc.)

What is the impact of missing the "ballgame" because you're so busy taking care of everyone else's needs?

Why do you keep "climbing the stairs" but not really getting anywhere?

If someone says to you, "What do you want?" are you ready to place your order?

(And no, I'm not talking about actual hot dogs, but if we were, I'd take one with mustard, an overpriced beer, and a solid view of the game.)

To the Lady with the Large Family – I think you're great. You clearly love your family, and you're willing to do anything for them. And you got a lot of exercise that day. (So did I, all that up-and-down to stand and let you pass.)

I'm just wondering what you might like to order if you could get anything you wanted on the Menu of Life.

Give it some thought.

You've got nine innings to live. Don't waste them fetching someone else's hot dog.

Play ball.

# CHAPTER 11

# THE STRIVING NARRATOR

## *More Is Never Enough*

The Striving Narrator is ambitious and believes there's always a better next chapter ahead. If you're a Striver, you believe in growth and doing the work to get there. Never satisfied, you push yourself to do more, be more, achieve more.

Sounds great, right?

The problem is the Striving Narrator is *always* striving. Rather than appropriately celebrating accomplishments, you're on to the next thing. You're never satisfied. No matter how well you do, that inner voice thinks you can do better. Got a 1570 on your SAT? Why not a 1600? Knocked two minutes off your 5k time? Keep working and maybe you can take off another two!

The Striving Narrator is someone for whom great isn't good enough. Strivers can work themselves to exhaustion and often feel unsatisfied. "What's next?" they ask. "I'm capable of more!"

If you find that you set and smash goals and that the satisfaction you gain is short lived, you might have a Striving Narrator, one that's telling you that you can never rest or be happy until you land at some future destination. It's like having a goal line that is being moved farther and farther away.

It can be exhausting. I once heard an Olympic gymnast give an interview during which she talked about her desire to continue training for four more years for the opportunity to earn a spot on another Olympic team. The workouts were grueling and hard on her body. She knew she might be doing long-term damage to her bones and joints. And yet, she couldn't stop striving. "It's like having a motor driving you on that you'd like to smash," is how I recall she described her ambition and desire.

You can only rev that motor so often before it burns out.

There are many ways we can grow. Yet, every so often you need to look at this great big mountain you're climbing and – rather than only looking ahead at how much farther you have to go – take a look back at how far you've already come. And reset the destination. Is that mountain peak the one you still want to climb?

## Tips to Silence a Striving Narrator:

- Stop. Pause. Reflect. Relish in the accomplishment before setting out for the next big goal.

- When someone thinks you're awesome, believe them! Don't negate your experiences simply because they are yours. Much like you admire someone else, try to see yourself through someone else's eyes.

- Don't dismiss compliments and accolades while only absorbing criticism. Consider what you hear and why. Why filter out the good stuff?

- Who is setting the expectations you want to reach? Where did they originate? Why does the finish line keep moving?

- Ask yourself, "When will it be enough? What does 'enough' look like?"

- Refine goals and adjust the course as necessary. For the goal-oriented among us, we're so focused on completing the task or reaching the next rung that we don't often stop to ask, "Is this still meaningful and worthwhile to me?"

- Recognize it doesn't all need to be done today, or at all. Including this list.

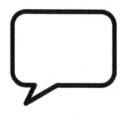

# CHAPTER 12

# NEXT STEPS

## *Now What?*

Now that we've reviewed 10 types of unreliable narrators, which ones resonate with you? Did you find yourself saying, "That sounds familiar!" Or "At least I don't hear *that* in my head!" Did it make you feel better to know you're not alone and that others suffer from a faulty, unreliable, or overly critical voice?

You may find you identify with one in particular or several narrators at once. You can see the challenges of each narrator, how they overlap, and how tips to control one narrator are applicable to others. Through the "Often/Sometimes/Never" framework introduced in Chapter 1, you can map your narrative type, the specific combination that shows up most frequently. For example, Squash is a Critical, Ruminating Striver (my "often"), who can be both a People Pleaser and an Arrogant ("sometimes") depending on the situation. If you move those words around and make an acronym, we find that Squash is full of CRAP(S).

Like Squash, your narrator is a combination of types gleaned from early experiences and polished and perfected from the perceptions of every single experience since. Where did that voice come from? What does it believe? Why is it there? Understanding that the narrator is a part of your experience but isn't the *actual* experience itself is even more important.

Acknowledging the critical or ruminating or self-centered thoughts in your head is the first step. The next one is: How to change it? How do we effectively "fire" that narrator and recast a more positive and productive voice in its place? That part is not quite as easy, but it can be done. It's like feeding yourself a steady diet of junk food knowing it's not good for you, and then, after much commitment, realizing the benefits of clean eating. We're going to clean up those thoughts in your head and address the mind garbage you feed yourself daily.

Want to dine on healthier fare? Like a variety of narrators, a variety of tips can alleviate the presence of unhelpful thoughts and clean up the narrative. Each of the following 10 chapters offers specific ways to address your thought process, reframe your experiences, and ultimately rewrite your story. You will find some that are easy to institute and provide immediate relief. Others may require more intentional practice. You will need to review your skepticism or pessimism or any other thoughts your narrator is already saying about your ability to improve and change.

Give it a try. What happens next is up to you.

# A STORY:
## Stop Feeding Yourself Garbage

You wouldn't eat it, would you?

It's bad for you.

Unhealthy.

Unsatisfying.

Toxic.

So why do you keep feeding yourself garbage?

I'm not talking about those Twinkies, Ding-Dongs, and Ho Ho's you keep tucked away in the pantry for the kids' school lunchboxes that somehow find their way into your mouth at 10 p.m. after a particularly stressful day.

I mean those thoughts you feed yourself. The ones with no nutritious value that leave you feeling lousy inside.

We serve our minds a daily diet and digest it even when we know we deserve better.

I hear it from clients all the time:

"I'm too old to try something new."

"This will never work."

"I feel totally stuck."

"I'm desperate to get a job."

"Everyone hates me."

Or, in the case of my friend "Jean," "I'm not good enough. Not smart enough. I missed out on the happiness and success that others have. It's too late for me."

Whoa.

And here's the thing about Jean – she has an amazing job in education where she has influenced the lives of thousands of students. She has an active social life and a long marriage. And she enjoys travel, theater, and martinis. Also, she's an amazing friend to many, and it pains me to think she'd ever see herself this way.

So where does all that crap come from?

The recesses of our overthinking, hypercritical, insecure minds are like a landfill.

Full of mind garbage.

What thoughts are you feeding yourself?

Is any of that mind garbage actually true?

Where does that voice come from? Why do you seem to have an insatiable appetite for what it offers?

Chew on that for a bit.

If your inner thoughts reek like something rotten, it's time to change up your diet. If you consistently ate a diet of garbage, you'd get sick. Why then would you feed your mind such garbage?

Time to trash those stinky thoughts and fill up on healthier ones. Here's my recommended daily allowance of better statements to fuel your motivation and feed your soul:

"I bring value wherever I go."

"Change is difficult, but it's possible."

"I have choices in every situation."

"I have people who know, trust, and support me."

"I am enough."

"My feelings are important and matter."

"The best is yet to come."

After all, you are what you eat.

Feed your thoughts appropriately.

Anything else belongs in the trash.

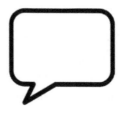

# CHAPTER 13

# IDENTIFY THE ORIGIN

## *Cruel Beginnings*

Understanding the genesis of your narrative thoughts – when and where they occurred in your past and why – is key to taking charge of them in your present. Consider the thought. What's your recollection of the messaging? Write it down. Who said it? What's the memory? Determine how that inner voice originated – whether it represents harsh words from childhood, a bullying boss, or a belittling old boyfriend. How did we somehow create the most critical of characters and put them in the most critical of roles? Get to the start of the story.

I can trace Squash back to my awkward teen years when I had braces and a bad perm and my biggest fear was two-fold. One, that no one would notice me. I'd go my entire life without ever making a mark, feeling successful, or hearing applause. And two, that someone might notice me. Talk about a Catch-22!

I wanted someone to notice me, but I didn't want them to notice me because what if they didn't like what they noticed? They might think I was not good enough. Not pretty enough or thin enough or smart enough or accomplished enough. So, I hid.

Squash took root. "You're not special," she'd say. Rude.

As if in response to that inner thought, I sought out ways to *be* special, trying to prove my own teen worthiness to myself. Freshman year I tried out for and made my high school ski team. And not only the varsity team, the A-team, the more competitive of the two varsity squads. Who wants to be on the B-team? Not me! I should probably point out that I was, at best, an intermediate skier with some speed. My high school in New York was much closer to the Bronx than it was to Lake Placid and not a hothouse of developing ski talent. (Here's Squash, making sure I let you know I was not actually a great skier, lest you momentarily presume so.)

I was proud of making the ski team, and to me, it was a big deal. It was a big enough deal that the school paper ran a small article about me. I remember briefly answering a student reporter's questions and the picture they snapped of me with my bad perm and mouth full of braces.

And I remember, vividly, the day the article came out. I saw my friends in the lunchroom hovered over the school paper. And there I was – bad perm and all – my photo with the caption of a quote from my interview: "While most freshmen start on the B-team, I made the A-team."

Had I said that? I suppose so. Had I said it *that way?* In black and white, it read differently than how I had meant it. But still, it was a nice article acknowledging my athletic achievement. I expected congratulations from my friends. Instead, the table was quiet. Until someone – I don't recall which friend, but it felt like group consensus – said, "You're so full of yourself. You shouldn't brag so much."

I don't remember what was said next. I do remember that I ate lunch alone that day. I had broken some unwritten girl code. "Thou shall not speak highly of thyself." And I was being punished for it. The cost of owning my special achievement was that I found myself alone.

What happened next? I made it all the way to the New York State high school ski sectionals where our little team from near the Bronx competed with schools that had mountains as their back-drop. There I had my top finish in the giant slalom – 32nd place. The following year, budget cuts at the school eliminated all fringe sports and took the ski team with it. And, with that, my high school ski career was done. These days, all that's left of it is watching my kids fly past me on a blue run and looking forward to après-ski at the bar when I can take my boots off and have a Bloody Mary.

Yet, years later, that moment in the lunchroom remains. It was a formative moment for Squash, one that followed me around and still pops up from time to time. Squash is there to remind me of the humiliation of eating alone in that lunchroom while striving to prove that I'm worthy. When I'm introduced at a keynote as a "ten-time Emmy-winning producer," something that is factually true, I struggle to own it. "You're so full of yourself," Squash whispers to me, in a voice that sounds much like one of those ninth-grade girls

I was once so close with. "You shouldn't brag so much."

When I speak about the impact of our inner narrator, I often use this moment as a real-life example. Yes, I'm standing on stage in front of you about to address my expertise on this topic. But that doesn't mean I'm not just as challenged by it as you are. I suffer from it too. I get it. I've spent decades unpacking stories in order to be able to reframe them.

Like me, you might need to go back in time to look for the story. When did it start? Who said it? What happened? Knowing the origins of the narrative helps put it into context so that you separate it from the present and don't carry it into the future.

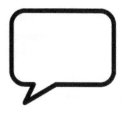

## CHAPTER 14

# DON'T FEAR FEAR

## *It's Just an "F" Word*

Would you believe that Squash isn't all bad? All of those criticisms, the second-guessing, the reminders of times gone wrong – she actually thinks she's doing me a favor!

Although it seems to serve no purpose, our inner narrator has one. Our narrative point of view is driven by vivid memories and powerful emotions like fear. Fear of not fitting in, of not being "enough," of failing others, or falling short of our own potential. Our inner narrators thrive on that fear as much as they seek to protect us from it. They feed us stories to keep us safe. Worried your idea might not be well received at the meeting? Your narrator will talk you out of offering it. Think you'll be rejected if you apply for that job? Maybe you shouldn't.

By naming the emotion, we can separate it from action. If it's fear, what do you fear? What worries you? Not achieving enough? Not being "special" enough? Not being liked? Why do you fear this? What's the worst that can happen? In what way is your narrator feeding into that fear, reiterating it, or trying to protect you from it? By attempting to protect us from what we fear, the narrator thinks it's keeping us safe. What it's really doing is making us stuck. When you understand why you are motivated by fear or how early experiences and messages have created the narrative point of view, you stop regarding that voice as truth.

Acknowledge the beneficial purpose of the voice and get to the root of the matter by considering the emotion behind the thought. Only then can you determine the best way to proceed.

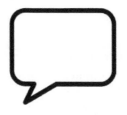

## CHAPTER 15

# EXAMINE THE EVIDENCE

## *Who Says It's So?*

*"To be persuasive, we must be believable; to be believable,*
*we must be credible; to be credible, we must be truthful."*
– Edward R. Murrow

I encourage everyone to be a journalist. You don't need formal training to fact-check statements like these: "I'm a big fat mess!" Or, "I'm never going to get promoted." Where's the evidence? Feelings aren't facts.

Stories tend to build upon themselves as we look for confirmation of our beliefs while disregarding evidence to the contrary. Your narrator does a great job functioning as a filter, flushing all thoughts that don't support its story.

When a thought pops into your head and you know it's Squash speaking, run the speech through a thorough fact-check.

Ask yourself:

Is it true?

Who says it's true?

What evidence is there that it's true?

What's the counterevidence that it's not?

If you spill your coffee at your desk and find your Squash saying, "You never do anything right!" where's all the evidence to the contrary? Consider all the times you drink your coffee without spilling (I'd guess there are many!) to remind yourself you are more than this one moment.

Next, analyze the cost of allowing yourself to believe the thought without questioning it. What's the impact of believing it? What's the benefit of questioning it? How does this particular thought fit into the big picture? I have too many clients who struggle to distinguish situational challenges from overarching flaws. Some even create and take ownership of full-blown personality defects out of them.

So you got salad dressing on your new shirt and then made the stain worse by trying to blot it out. Sounds like a messy situation. It does not mean you're always a "mess." Yelling at your kids doesn't make you a "bad mom," sleeping in one day doesn't make you permanently "lazy," not getting the job doesn't make you a "loser," etc.

Don't let your inner narrator create permanent, unflattering labels just because telemarketing calls infuriate you or you accidentally cut the extension power cord with the hedge trimmer. (I did that once, and clearly, I should have been more careful in that particular circumstance.)

Consider "Brooke," who was so nervous the night before her presentation that she could barely sleep. She combatted her fatigue with an extra cup of coffee at breakfast and then felt jittery and sweaty when it was time to take the stage. Brooke's performance was worse in her own head than it was to anyone in the audience, but that didn't stop her from judging herself harshly. "I'm just not a good public speaker," she concluded. "I don't have the confidence. What's the point in even doing this? All the other speakers were so much better."

In this case, Brooke took the specific circumstances (anxiety + lack of sleep + extra caffeine + jitters + feeling uncomfortable on stage) and came to the conclusion that her public speaking skills – in fact, her entire sense of confidence – were flawed. Wouldn't anyone be nervous in that type of situation? Why evaluate yourself without considering the circumstances surrounding the action?

Together we were able to examine the evidence, which thankfully included a video recording so that she could see proof of her more-than-solid presentation and how her inner concerns weren't outwardly visible. We then worked on taming her very Critical, Runaway, Defeatist Narrator.

Another way to examine the evidence is to consider the consequences of the thoughts. Even if the statement is true, what's the impact? Let's say I'm running late for an appointment, but I really need my coffee, so I stop at Dunkin' on the way. I'm in line, and the woman in front of me not only doesn't know what she wants but is asking the cashier about the caloric count for each donut so that she can pick the healthiest option. I'm late and undercaffeinated and annoyed, and it's taking every bit of my self-control to not yell, "They're donuts, lady!"

And then I feel bad because why can't I just be a more patient person, unperturbed by small, inconsequential moments such as these? Why do I tap my foot and roll my eyes and audibly sigh until I get my coffee and am safely back in my car? Later, after some reflection, I no longer feel irritated at the nice lady who wanted a low-calorie donut. I feel ashamed. I berate myself for not being a more patient human being. Squash tells me I should have handled it differently, that I'm always like this, that I'm a bad person.

You likely have your own version of this story. Why not ask yourself this question instead: "So what?" So what if I was overly impatient in an otherwise inconsequential moment? So what if I'm the type of person who gets irritated when the person at the donut shop is seeking a low-calorie donut, and I find that *absolutely ridiculous?*

That makes me human, not horrible. And then I can follow up with, "Now what?" This puts the control back in my hands. Now that this has happened, what do I want to do next? Do I want to use it as motivation to become a more patient person? Do I want to familiarize myself with the nutritional content of all the donuts so that I can be a more helpful bystander the next time this happens? Or do I just want to let it go as a single frustrating experience and not have it be indicative of some overarching character flaw?

Examine the evidence. Ask yourself what matters. Decide what you want to do (differently) the next time. And, in case you're wondering, the lowest calorie donut at Dunkin' is the French cruller.[6] Now you know and won't need to hold up the line for the answer.

---

[6] Hurrah, donut lovers! You can save 150 calories by ordering that French cruller (230 calories) instead of the multi-grain bagel (380 calories)! https://www.dunkindonuts.com/en/menu/nutrition

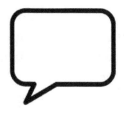

## CHAPTER 16

# NAME IT TO
# SEPARATE IT

## *Your Evil Alter Ego*

Squash. Sally. Shithead.

Does your inner narrator have a name? Squash would like to make her acquaintance. My friend Louise, an excellent leadership and life coach, calls her inner voice Sally. She says when Sally gets to be a particular nuisance, she tells Sally to go to the corner. We've joked that Squash and Sally could author an entire series of books.

*Squash and Sally Ruin Your Day!*

*Squash and Sally Feel Out of Shape at the Gym!*

*Squash and Sally's Vacation Accompanied by Daily Rain!*

If you haven't already named your narrator, I suggest you do.

Besides allowing you an opportunity for levity and humor, the process serves to separate the thoughts from who you truly are. Squash is not Valerie; I know that. Squash is a small part of me that continues to squash the real me and the potential of the future me. There are studies that show that simply referring to yourself in the third person allows you to more objectively approach circumstances.[7]

Thinking of your narrator as an entirely separate character in the story, one that is clearly different from your hero or heroine (a reminder – if you need it – that's *you!*), helps you think of it as its own entity. The narrator is the evil villain you fight to get to the resolution of the story, your "happily ever after." Giving your narrator a name, like my Squash, can bring objectivity to your own thinking and allow you to "talk back." (This sounds odder than it is unless, of course, you engage in such dialogue out loud and in the middle of your busy day.)

Once you've named your narrator, you've effectively separated it from your evidence-based thinking. Also, it's funny to name this character and give it a distinct personality. Like Squash, the Viking Russian squash-like object. Like Sally, a petulant child who needs to be sent to the corner. Like Larry, who is so worried about being a loser that he won't even get in the game.

What do you want to name your narrator? Make it one that suits her. Karen. Ken. Helga the Horrible. Dipshit. And then tell it to shut up.

---

[7] There's psychology behind it and another book you should read that Squash says is better than this one! https://www.psychologytoday.com/us/blog/the-novel-perspective/201506/fooling-your-ego

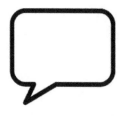

## CHAPTER 17

# STAY IN THE PRESENT

## *Be Here Now*

Squash is a unique combination of narrator styles, including the Ruminator and the Striver. The Ruminator keeps me rooted in the past with too much attention to "shoulda, woulda, coulda" and "if only I knew then what I know now." The Striver keeps me firmly future-focused and living in search of unreached goals.

Where do I rarely find myself? In the present! Because our narrator reflects so strongly on interpretation of past experiences and spends the rest of the time worrying about the as-of-yet-unwritten future, it's rarely living in the present. It seems its present role is to keep us stuck in the past and fearful of the future.

Knowing my tendency to ruminate and strive, I've had to practice being present and mindful in the moment. It's such an unfamiliar place for me that I knew I'd need help to even figure out how to do it. Out of curiosity and a dogged determination (hello, Striver!), I enrolled in an eight-week mindfulness stress reduction course. I showed up as a Striver ("I must get better at this!") while also Adamant that it was a waste of time. ("This is never going to work!") In fact, I showed up not only skeptical, but somewhat resistant to the entire process.

I explained to the instructor, a calm woman who I was certain was judging me, that a friend had scoffed when she heard I had enrolled in the course. What she said was, "You can't turn a racehorse into a turtle." I had to admit my friend's assessment was spot on. Not only am I a racehorse, always ready to go, I *like* being a racehorse. Did I have to change? Who was I to think I could become a turtle, content to move at a slower pace?

"So be a racehorse," the instructor advised. "Be a racehorse but be here." She wasn't trying to turn me into a turtle. She was welcoming of racehorses. We were to show up exactly as we were without judgment or worry.

Without judgment? Isn't that what our very judgy narrators are always trying to do? But I was determined to try to quiet the narrator within me telling me I had wasted money on a course I clearly wouldn't like.

During the first class, I thought I was going to jump out of my skin. I was literally itchy. The silence and stillness were excruciating. And I was quickly frustrated with myself. Why did my mind wander so quickly and so frequently? Were the other attendees thinking as much as I was? Why is this so hard? What should I make for dinner? Are we out of mayonnaise? WHY am I thinking about mayo?

And so it went. Week after week of my attempting to sit in stillness and find my mind wandering. Anywhere. Everywhere. I asked the instructor – what was wrong with me? She reminded me that mindfulness is a practice. That's why they call it a practice! The only way to do it "wrong" is to not do it at all.

Did it get easier over time? Yes. Do I still do it "wrong," noticing my thoughts wandering to past and present? Yep, every time. But what I did find was the more I practiced this stillness, the better I felt afterwards and the more I looked forward to the next session. On days I skipped the practice, I didn't feel as good. This convinced me that my efforts, though often racing and seemingly "wrong," were indeed worth it.

In time, I learned to stay present, and I practice that mindfulness multiple times daily, sometimes only for a breath or two. It's like hitting the reset button on the Ruminating and Striving brain. Hey, we're here now. We're not in the past, feeling foolish or remorseful. We're not in the future, focused on some next-level goal. We are here.

Be here now.

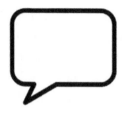

CHAPTER 18

# UNPACK THE CART

## *What Are You Carrying Around?*

I went into the store to get two items. How many did I come out with? (Hint: the store is Target.) If you're unfamiliar with this big-box shopping destination, substitute one in your town. You know the kind of store I mean. The one where you go in for two items and come out with a cart full of stuff a wallet that's $200 lighter.

For some reason, I can't emerge from Target without spending the equivalent of a small mortgage payment. There's just so much there that I need or think I need or know I'll need some day. And the carts are so big! So much space to add items. On this particular day, my plan was to purchase a desk lamp and bulletin board for my daughter's room so she could set up a study station. That's it. Two items.

I found the lamp. In fact, I found two after deciding my son needed one as well. I didn't find the bulletin board in the right size, so I headed to check out. On the way there, I realized my nephew's birthday was coming up, so I might as well get him a gift now, and grab a card and some wrapping paper. We can always use tissues and toilet paper – why not stock up now? And is it double-A or triple-A batteries we're always low on? Better get both. Some cans of seltzer, snacks – ooh, look, a neutral eye palette, and it's on sale...

Finally, I make it to the checkout lane and the friendly cashier asks me in that chipper way, as they always do, "Did you find everything you were looking for?"

And I look in my cart, at the desk lamp I planned to buy (and the one I didn't) buried under a mass of items. Who put those Doritos in there? And I say to her, honestly, "No. But I found a lot of stuff I wasn't looking for!"

I head out to the parking lot to load my newly purchased items into my car. The shopping cart, now full, is heavy and unwieldy, and I have difficulty navigating the curb and divots in the sidewalk. I'm steering and pushing and that's when I realize – all this stuff in my cart – some of which I need and is helpful and most of which is not – is now mine. And it's heavy. And unwieldy. And I'm wondering why I need any of it.

Let me stop to ask you the pressing question here:

What's in your cart?

I don't mean your cart at Target (though I'm curious if it's as full as mine); I mean all this "stuff" – these stories – that you've collected over the years, which seemed necessary or helpful at the time, that you continue to carry around with you.

That "stuff" is heavy. Does it still serve you?

What might we learn from how we fill our carts? What might happen if we unpack the cart, examine what's inside, and keep only what's most useful now?

If you want to fill your cart with more of what you need and less of what you don't (no more mind garbage!), ask yourself some of the following questions:

Why am I holding on to this thought?

Is there value in this story?

How is this serving me?

How have I grown since this happened?

What is still true?

How might I use this information?

Does this matter?

What can I let go of?

Who do I want to be ... now?

Empty the cart of all past stories. Examine them for evidence. Question them. Don't just wheel them around for years, wondering why they are yours. There's a cost to owning them, and it's more than what you spend while running errands at Target.

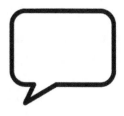

CHAPTER 19

# SWITCH THE PERSPECTIVE

## *Best Friend vs. Worst Critic*

Are you your own best friend? Or your worst critic?

Those things you say to yourself – would you ever say them to someone you care about? If your narrator sounds more like your worst critic than your best friend, it's time to get a better voice. (This is the point when I remind you that if your best friend and your worst critic are the *same* person, it's time for a new best friend!)

Let's play devil's advocate to get at that devil of a voice. Let's take the opposite approach, a complete 180, and see what it sounds like. So, if your voice says that not landing the job you interviewed for is because you're never going to get one, try switching the perspective and saying the exact opposite. For example, "I will get a job that's right for me." Or, if you're criticizing yourself for falling off your diet again, and you think you can't do anything right, switch the perspective. "I can succeed at many things."

If this all sounds a little too much like Stuart Smalley from *Saturday Night Live* ("I'm good enough, I'm smart enough, and gosh darn it, people like me!"), consider that positive mantras have a place in generating motivation and energy. Plus, they make you feel good!

If that's too much of a switch for you, go back to your fact-checking to neutralize the statement. "I'm disappointed to not get this job, but it's not the only one I can apply for." "I broke my commitment to my diet, but I can focus on healthy eating again whenever I choose."

Switching the perspective, whether it's to a more positive voice (your inner cheerleader) or an objective one (your inner journalist), stops the original and unhelpful thought from gaining momentum.

You want things to be different? Start by thinking differently.

# A STORY:
# The Party in Your Head
# You Didn't Intend to Host

They show up without warning and stay too long. You've probably hosted such an event, unintentionally and reluctantly. And yet, it's hard to show them the door. Because there's no obvious exit when the venue is your busy brain. Let's set the scene:

Where: My bedroom

When: 3:00 a.m.

ANXIETY: Hiiii! You up?

ME: Huh ... what?

ANXIETY: Want to think about how much you have to do tomorrow?

ME: Umm, no, I was just sleeping.

ANXIETY: How about mulling over a bunch of things that are highly unlikely to happen but would be really tragic if they did?

ME: What? No!

ANXIETY: Oh, OK. Let me just ask a question. Did you shut the garage door before you went to bed?

ME: Yes.

ANXIETY: You sure?

ME: ... I think so –

ANXIETY: Maybe you should check. Thieves could get in. A bear. A skunk. It's probably open.

UNNECESSARILY HARSH CRITIC: You always forget everything!

ME: Who are you?

ANXIETY: Oh, I brought some friends. You remember them.

UNNECESSARILY HARSH CRITIC: I'm back!

RUMINATION: Me too! Want to review every foolish thing you ever did?

ME: I need to sleep. I have to get up early for work.

ANXIETY: Oh, right, it's Presentation-in-Front-of-Important-People Day!

UNNECESSARILY HARSH CRITIC: You're going to blow it.

ME: What? Why?

UNNECESSARILY HARSH CRITIC: Because you suck.

ME: Hang on, wait … at what?

UNNECESSARILY HARSH CRITIC: At everything.

ANXIETY: Now that we're all here hanging out, let's get that heart rate up!

RUMINATION: Remember last time you gave a presentation the PowerPoint didn't advance? And you were stuck on that same slide forever?

ME: Ugh. That was awful.

RUMINATION: I know, right? So embarrassing! Let's relive it in full detail.

ME: Please, no. I have to go back to sleep.

ANXIETY: Ooh, it's racing – we've got a racing heart!

UNNECESSARILY HARSH CRITIC: You never take care of yourself. You're going to look all puffy tomorrow.

RUMINATION: Just like last week when you went out for a glass of wine and drank the bottle.

UNNECESSARILY HARSH CRITIC: You're fat.

ANXIETY: Hey, it's a party! Let me play an entirely annoying song over and over again. How about that '90s classic "Mmm Bop" by Hansen?

ME: No! That's a terrible song.

ANXIETY: Here we go! "Mmmbop, ba duba dop, ba du bop, duba dop!" I'll just put it on repeat, so it stays with you for a while.

ME: Stop! That's not even how the song goes.

UNNECESSARILY HARSH CRITIC: Your taste in music sucks.

RUMINATION: Just like that time you got caught with the window down singing out loud to *NSYNC. And that guy in the other car looked at you really funny. Remember? "It might sound crazy, but it ain't no lie – Baby, bye bye bye!"

ANXIETY: Wow, you're sweating. And your heart is going so fast! Does it feel like it might explode? It might explode. That would be bad.

UNNECESSARILY HARSH CRITIC: Did I mention you suck?

- END SCENE -

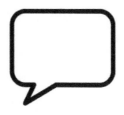

## CHAPTER 20

# REPLACE THE EMOTION

## *Feel Better Feels*

Our narrators have a funny way of showing up unannounced at inopportune times. Sometimes they come with friends, equally unhelpful party guests who create chaos instead of fun. The result is too many words and opinions, few of them helpful, all of them creating noise, confusion, self-doubt, and fatigue.

How do you ward off uninvited guests? If you're going to have company, especially the kind that takes up space *in your head,* you'll need to be particular about who gets an invite. When you fill the space with better guests – the ones you really want to spend time with – then those you don't want will have less room to make themselves comfortable and maybe won't show up at all.

Use what you've learned in any situation to create more

successful scenes moving forward. Rather than beating yourself up over something gone wrong, embrace the information as knowledge helpful for the next go-round.

What if we calmed our thoughts with a steady infusion of more positive emotions? Much like switching the perspective from worst critic to best friend, try swapping out unhelpful emotions for better ones.

Some to consider:

**Gratitude.** What are you thankful for?

**Authenticity.** Congratulate yourself for being a real and honest human being with fears and failings.

**Community.** Accepting yourself and showing up as you truly are makes you more relatable. You'll find you're not in this alone. There are plenty of others who feel just like you do.

**Optimism.** Instead of focusing on what might go wrong, think about what is going well and what might continue to go well in the future.

**Big-picture thinking.** What matters in the long run?

**Joy.** Did you know you are allowed to enjoy yourself? What small things might make a difference in your daily life?

**Humor.** It's kind of funny you let this make-believe person in your head feed you such nonsense.

We are the company we keep. So, keep control of who accompanies you. Edit your guest list – even the one to the fictional party in your head – accordingly.

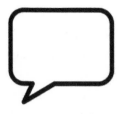

# CHAPTER 21

# CASTING CALL

## *Recast That Role*

Now that we've identified the origins and questioned and replaced the thoughts and emotions that feed our inner narrator, we're ready to hold a casting call. You're the director of this show in your head. You can replace your narrator with a more beneficial version. Who should play the part? Perhaps Glinda the Good Witch telling you, "You've always had the power, my dear. You just had to learn it for yourself."

By simply substituting two letters with one, I can cast an entirely new narrator. Take the *sh* off the end of Squash and add a *d*, and now I've got "Squad." When I think of the squad I'd much prefer to accompany me, I get an image in my head of those fierce and focused Wakandan warriors from the *Black Panther* movie. That's who I'd want by my side, watching my back. Why not put them in my head?

If you're someone who finds your narrator tends to gang up on you, you need a new gang! What might it look like to have a healthy narrator? Replace the image, rewrite the voice, and recast your narrator. Much as you created a name for the faulty voice in your head, give this newly cast version an identity. It's the superhero in you. It *is* you. Bring your new narrator to life and let it narrate life's difficult moments.

In no time at all, your Squad will squash your Squash..

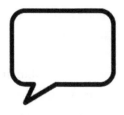

## CHAPTER 22

# WATCH YOUR LANGUAGE

## *Red Flag Words*

How do you know when your inner narrator is at play? It tends to use language that's one-sided, overly pessimistic, or very black and white. Recognize when these red flag words arise and call attention to them. (Fact-check! Switch the perspective!)

What words should we listen for?

**Too.** Too is a red flag word when it's used as a judgment. How often have we felt "too" (much/little) to be good enough? "I'm too old," you might think, as you consider going back to school. Or,

"I'm too inexperienced," as you consider applying for the role. We're "too loud," "too opinionated," or "too fat to go to the gym." And these are too, too many judgments.

**Should.** If you find yourself thinking you "should" (or shouldn't) have done something or behaved a certain way, your narrator is making a judgment about your behavior. And although it's great to have high standards and expectations for yourself, if you have a Critic or Striver narrator, you're probably "should-ing" on yourself a lot.

Replace your should with could for a more objective take. You should have gone to the gym? You *could* have gone to the gym, but you chose not to. You should have kept quiet instead of correcting your boss? You *could* have kept quiet. You have options in all of your actions. You could choose to do this – or that. Should you? That's up to you.

**Always/Never.** Ah, the two dominant phrases of the Adamant Narrator. If you find you are always thinking about always and never, you're likely viewing your world in a very black-and-white, all-or-nothing manner. Try imparting a little flexibility with more flexible words such as *usually*, *typically*, *preferably*, etc.

**If only.** Defeatist narrators love "if only" because it makes them think their current circumstances are unlikely to change so why bother with effort? "If only" speaks to past disappointments, missed opportunities, and less-than-ideal circumstances that keep us from living our best lives. If only we could move on from our "if only" to ask, "What if?"

**Just.** Don't we like things that are just? Not when we're not doing ourselves justice! Just give me a minute because I've got something to say. You need a big adjustment. You have a "just" problem. You know the "just" I'm talking about – the one you insert into conversation when it has no reason to be there.

I ask, "So, what do you do?" And you reply, "I'm just a mom," or "I'm just an assistant." I say, "Tell me about yourself," and you sheepishly admit, "I'm just not that interesting." I congratulate you on the well-run event, and you shrug and offer, "I'm just a volunteer." You pepper your emails with this phrase: "Just checking in!" as if offering an apology.

If only we could just stop adding just as a qualifying statement! Why do we justify our existence with just? What justification is there for doing so? How does it help? You need to stop "just-ifying" yourself.

Instead of answering "What do you do?" with "I'm just a mom" or "I'm just a volunteer," say it without such justification:

"I'm busy raising my family."

"I'm volunteering on the board raising money for the school."

And instead of justifying your action with any sort of an unnecessary preamble ("I'm just checking in with you," "I just have a question"), complete the action, ask the question, do the thing without worrying about what other people might think! It's (just) that simple.

While we're focused on identifying those red flag words, consider the wordiness we often use before our words, that lengthy preamble that kills our message. I'm talking about our need to give explanation before the statement and how, by doing so, we often shoot ourselves in the foot before we even get started.

I'm talking about the hedge. I know it might sound silly, but it's one of my pet peeves. It's probably not a big deal in the grand scheme of things, but it just bugs me sometimes. You might not be bothered by it, but I am...

Are you wondering when I'm going to get to the point? That's what happens when people hedge, saying all sorts of *other* stuff before they get to the good stuff, and in doing so, diminishing their argument or statement before they've had the chance to make it.

Why do we hedge our statements by including in them the very thing we *don't* want to hear? It's as if we're hedging our bets. We presume that if we say it first, we'll have addressed the concern we think others already have. The problem is that it puts our concern – the very thing we want to avoid – right in front of our audience!

According to Etymology Online, the phrase "hedge your bets" dates back to the 1600s and originated from the concept of planting a hedge to enclose and protect a piece of land.[8] The hedge reduces the risk of harm, just as people hedge their bets at the casino or sports book, betting the opposite of their original bet to ensure a profit. Like how hedge funds invest in both long and short stocks to protect against market fluctuations. Like how hedgehogs – oh, never mind. Hedgehogs have nothing to do with this. But they sure are cute.

---

[8] Sourced from https://www.etymonline.com/. You learn cool stuff like this when you write a book that makes you a lot of fun at parties.

You know what's not a helpful hedge? The unnecessary preamble. If you're trying to protect against potential rejection or ridicule, why would you spoon-feed your audience the very things you want to avoid? If you have something to say, say it.

Confidently. Convincingly. Compellingly. Conversationally. And, most importantly, concisely.

The exposition – or set-up – of a statement should exist only to give necessary or appropriate context. It shouldn't take away from the content itself.

Here are three examples of Horrible Hedging:

1. An attendee takes the mic during a conference Q&A:

"I have a silly question you've probably been asked a million times before...."

What's the question? Is it truly a silly question? Have I been asked it a million times? Now I'm wondering what the asker is wondering and find my mind wandering when it should be focused on listening. Most likely I'll offer the obligatory reply, "That's not a silly question," or "There are no silly questions."

Just. Ask. The. Question.

2. An employee raises her hand at the brainstorming meeting:

"This is probably a stupid idea, but ..."

NO, NO, NO! Don't say that. No one wants to hear your stupid idea. If it's truly a stupid idea, then go back to the drawing board.

If it's *not* a stupid idea, but you're afraid other people might *think* it is, why would you put the possibility that it's stupid in their heads before you even get a chance to find out if it's stupid? I mean, talk about stupid. That's stupid!

Just. Offer. The. Idea. Stand up for what you want to say. If you discover it's not a good idea, you'll either defend it or drop it and deliver another even better one.

3. A job candidate points out her lack of qualification in a cover letter:

"Though I only have three of the four years of experience you require for this role ..."

If you want the job, why would you start with reasons why they shouldn't give it to you? Rather than offering shortcomings, cite the experience and skills and attributes you possess. ("In my three years at Corporation X, I grew our sales profits x%.")

When we're worried someone won't like what we're offering, we think acknowledging potential issues up front will better convince them. But by putting those fears front and center, we might be creating an issue where there wasn't one to begin with.

The solution? Cut it out. Lose the preamble. Don't let your narrator make you think it's necessary. Just ask the question. Offer the idea. Apply for the job. You want to take root, grow, and flower? Trim that hedge. Watch what you say.

Words matter. Use ones that say you matter too.

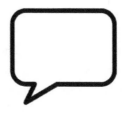

## CHAPTER 23

# ACTIVE AUTHORSHIP

## *Craft the Future Story*

*"Listen to your gut and follow your heart
but take your brain with you."*
– Commander-in-She

Now that you can recognize the many ways your narrator is unreliable and you have the tools to check this voice, what next? We've gotten to this present moment; what would you like to happen in the future? Are you going to take Squash with you and let her continue to squash you every day?

This is where you need to compartmentalize thought from action, so that you don't stay stuck in unhelpful thoughts from the past. If you want to craft a (better!) future story, start rewriting the next chapter. It takes practice. Here are a few remaining tips to edit your thoughts and flip that internal script.

**Talk Back.** Sometimes I get riled up and take Squash on. She sat on my shoulder during a run the other day and had something to say every step of the way. "You're so slow," she noted. "Why are you even out here? It's so hot. You should just stop." And I'd had enough of Squash. "Squash!" I yelled (a quiet yell to myself so as not to freak out any passersby), "You're not helping!" And then I proceeded to remind myself in a voice that is very much *mine*, "You're out here doing it. Just keep going. You're going to finish. Keep it up!" It didn't make me any faster or less sweaty. But it did make me feel better.

**Plan for the optimal outcome.** A negative narrator wants you to plan for failure and have a backup plan in place. Those thoughts of "if this doesn't work out, I can always ..." serve as safeguards but can also hold you back. If your plans don't materialize, you have plan B ready to go, your backup plan. Plan B is for when things go awry, or you don't get the *yes* or you run out of funds. How will you survive? What will you do next? Disaster awaits!

When I left my corporate job to launch my own company, my plan B included things like returning to the work I had done for more than 20 years, downsizing to reduce expenses, or getting an hourly job to pay the bills if my new line of work was not successful. I'd see hiring signs at Whole Foods and think, OK, well, I could always do that. Plan B was always on my mind, so much so that along with it, I added a plan C, a plan D, and a variety of other ways I would cope if I failed along the way – almost as if I was planning for failure.

Why do we plan for failure? Why didn't I give equal attention to what would happen if I not only succeeded in my first year of business but got all that I wanted and *more*? What if I achieved not only plan A, but a type of plan A++ I had never even dared to dream? Was I prepared for it to all work out?

What about you? What if it all works out *better* than you could have imagined? Let your narrator feed on that. Why would you not consider that possibility? Deep down you believe in yourself, but you let the voices of self-doubt tell you otherwise, so much so that when you picture the future, you plan for what might go wrong rather than what could go right. And you follow that narrative with a cautious, even pessimistic, approach. You're more likely to think that you won't get what you want than that you will. Your desire to protect yourself, to plan for what could happen if you don't get what you want, holds you back from considering what happens if you *do* get it all – and then some! Plan for success.

If success doesn't come, there will always be a plan B. But don't *plan* for the plan B. Plan for A+. You won't know what it looks like if you can't envision it. And you certainly won't be prepared if you don't plan for it.

**Compartmentalize thought from action.** Not feeling it? Proceed anyway. Neutralize the thought, swap the emotion for a better one, and don't let yourself get stuck in the past. Action is the antidote to anxiety. As Sir Isaac Newton discovered, objects in motion tend to stay in motion. Small steps matter. Small goals add up to big goals. Although I know some people who have crafted impressive 180-degree turns in life, most of us are more comfortable with incremental change. You don't need to quit your job, sell all your worldly possessions, and move to a tropical island to sell mangoes out of a hut in order to change your life for the better. (If that's truly your thing, go for it, but may I suggest checking visa requirements first?)

Remember that your past story – those choices you've made and actions you've taken – have created your present. Your present story – the choices you make now and actions you take daily – will create your future story. If you want a different story, start with the one you tell yourself inside your head. Your unhelpful inner narrator has played a role in your past. Don't let your narrator hijack your future. If you can neutralize and compartmentalize your thoughts, you won't carry them as an underlying narrative. In order to get unstuck, you have to take a step forward. You can't craft the future story without some forward motion. The key to creating a successful and satisfying next chapter is to serve as its active author.

This takes practice. Daily practice. Challenging, difficult, at times seemingly impossible practice. But it can be done.

At first, the changes may seem so small that you don't even notice them. Ultimately, what you are doing is creating minor edits and tiny trims to the story. These small changes will add up to big results. If you can replace your narrator, you can reframe your narrative point of view and the way you look at the world. If you can reframe your narrative point of view, you can rewrite the story. Every day is an opportunity to remove what no longer matters, serves, or grows you, and to add what does. Every day is an opportunity to turn the page and start with a blank sheet of paper. Fill it with what matters most to you.

It's your story. What happens next?

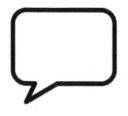

## CHAPTER 24

# YOUR (FINAL) NARRATOR CHECKLIST

## *Know More, Do Better*

- Identify which narrative types show up most frequently (Often/Sometimes/Never):

    The Critical Narrator

    The Runaway Narrator

    The Overthinking Narrator

    The Arrogant Narrator

    The Self-Centered Narrator

The Ruminating Narrator

The Adamant Narrator

The Defeatist Narrator

The People-Pleasing Narrator

The Striving Narrator

- Acknowledge your inner narrator is unreliable.

- Consider the origins of the story you tell yourself.

- Name the emotion that is driving the thought.

- Process the concern.

- Determine if the story is true.

- Consider when and how the story began.

- Put a name to who says it's true.

- Fact-check.

- Recognize the impact.

- Accentuate the positive.

- Switch the perspective.

- Neutralize the statement.

- Compartmentalize thought from action.

- Allow for compliments to complement criticisms.

- Talk back to your narrator (and argue if you have to!).

- Beware of red flag words like always and never.

- Don't get stuck in the past.

- Take action, the antidote to anxiety.

- Be open to learning and discovery.

- Plan for the optimal outcome.

- Consider there's no one right to way to do things.

- Craft the future story.

- Allow yourself to be human. (But don't spit on a donut if you can avoid doing so.)

# EPILOGUE

## STUFF IT, SQUASH!

Squash insisted that I'd never finish this book. With her on my shoulder and in my head, it took me longer than intended. But I made it. I finished. It's done.

But … maybe no one will buy it. Or read it. Or like it. Why did I even write it? Has anyone seen the Wheat Thins?

Stuff it, Squash!

# ACKNOWLEDGMENTS:

Writing a book isn't easy. It's even harder when you have a voice in your head that tells you it's a bad idea, you'll never finish it, that sentence makes no sense, etc., as Squash so often told me. So, I'm extra thankful for all the people who saw the best version of me and of this book even when I had trouble seeing that myself.

When I left my corporate career in 2017 to launch Commander-in-She, I walked away not just from what I was doing but who I was. I had this crazy idea that I'd figure out what I wanted to do and who I was meant to be. What started as an inkling for a single workshop became a full-fledged business. The first time I spoke of it was to my friend Julia Avery in a crowded bar. As I walked her through the workshop concept, she interrupted. "I love you," she said. Not that she loved the idea, which is what she meant, but that she loved me for putting the idea out there. To be fair, we had consumed a decent amount of vodka at that point, but it was the first time I thought, "Hmm, maybe I do have something here."

I remember when I described what would become my signature workshop, "What's Your Story?" to Tobi Libbra and she said,

"You know this is going to be really big, right?" I hadn't known that, but hearing that she believed it made me consider the possibility that it just might.

These are just two stories among many others from those who encouraged and supported me in those early years. Eventually their voices overtook the doubting one in my head.

This book was the natural extension of the "Recast Your Narrator, Rewrite Your Life" workshop. To all the attendees of the early offerings, especially Lauren Seder, Rich Fella, Fay Greenfield, Matt Maranz, and Teri Carden, thank you for walking through the material with me.

A huge shout-out to the ever-present supporting characters in this crazy story of mine: Mary Ellen Ladieu, Caryn Sullivan, Kelly Kennedy, Jessica Herzberg, and René Syler.

Thank you to Susan Rooks, the Grammar Goddess, for your keen eye and corrections and for reading and proofing my drafts. Thank you, Sarah Elkins for the introduction to Susan and for all your story support and inspiration. To the original sleepover crew - Anne, Deedre, Teri, Maggie, Jody, Tammy, Wendy, Ginger - how is it I feel I know you and you know me so well already? And to Teri, again, for the introduction to Erik Minder who helped translate my concept into the start of a book cover. Good people know good people.

To my early readers - Nisreen Cain, Louise Reid, Sara Nasshan, Christine Wilt, Shailavi Jain, Mary Ellen Ladieu - your feedback not only made the book better, it made me believe there was actually a book here! Thanks to my mom, my biggest cheerleader, for reading an early version, catching some errors, and agreeing the topic was necessary and worthwhile. She deserves an inner narrator who cheers her on the way she cheers for me.

My gratitude to my former CBS colleague Ashley Bernardi, for the introduction to Julie Broad and the Book Launchers team, and to Jaqueline Kyle, Melissa Sobey, and Nicole Larsen for helping me get this book over the finish line without getting Squashed.

Thank you to fellow authors who have inspired me with your beautiful words and wonderful ideas.

Finally, a big shout out to my family. My inner Squash often rears her ugly head out loud. Know that I want to do and be better for all of you.

Since Squash is screaming, "You know you're gonna forget someone, you dummy!" my sincere thanks to those I've neglected to mention here.

And my thanks to you, my reader. I hope this book helps make a difference in that all-important story in your head. Your success story starts there. Be its active author.

CPSIA information can be obtained
at www.ICGtesting.com
Printed in the USA
BVHW081323121021
618739BV00004B/62

9 781737 434504